COPING WITH CANCER STRESS

COPING WITH CANCER STRESS

edited by

BASIL A. STOLL
Honorary consultant physician to oncology departments
St. Thomas' Hospital and Royal Free Hospital
London, U.K.

Introduction by

AVERY D. WEISMAN
Professor of Psychiatry
Massachusetts General Hospital and Harvard Medical School
Boston, U.S.A.

1986 **MARTINUS NIJHOFF PUBLISHERS**
a member of the KLUWER ACADEMIC PUBLISHERS GROUP
DORDRECHT / BOSTON / LANCASTER

Distributors

for the United States and Canada: Kluwer Academic Publishers, 190 Old Derby Street, Hingham, MA 02043, USA
for the UK and Ireland: Kluwer Academic Publishers, MTP Press Limited, Falcon House, Queen Square, Lancaster LA1 1RN, UK
for all other countries: Kluwer Academic Publishers Group, Distribution Center, P.O. Box 322, 3300 AH Dordrecht, The Netherlands

Library of Congress Cataloging in Publication Data

```
Coping with cancer stress.

   Includes index.
   1. Cancer--Psychological aspects.  2. Stress
(Psychology)  3. Adjustment (Psychology)  I. Stoll,
Basil A. (Basil Arnold)  [DNLM: 1. Adaptation,
Psychological.  2. Neoplasms--psychology.  3. Stress,
Psychological.  QZ 200 C7837]
RC262.C635   1986      616.99'4'0019      85-21771
```

ISBN 0-89838-817-1

Contributors

Kerry Bluglass, M.B., Ch.B., M.R.C. Psych.
Consultant Psychiatrist, The Woodbourne Clinic, Birmingham; Senior Research
Fellow, Medical School, University of Birmingham, U.K.

Thurston B. Brewin, F.R.C.P., F.R.C.R.
Director, Institute of Radiotherapeutics and Oncology, Glasgow; Consultant to
Belvidere Hospital and Western Infirmary, Glasgow, U.K.

Robert Buckman, M.B., B. Chir., M.R.C.P.
Consultant Oncologist, Toronto-Bayview Clinic, Sunnybrook Medical Centre,
Toronto, Canada

Alan Coates, M.D., F.R.A.C.P.
Senior Specialist in Medical Oncology, Ludwig Institute for Cancer Research;
Medical Oncologist, Royal Prince Alfred Hospital, Sydney, Australia

Alastair J. Cunningham, Ph.D.
Professor, Department of Medical Biophysics, University of Toronto; Member
of Senior Scientific Staff, Ontario Cancer Institute, Toronto, Canada

K. De Meij,
Health Educator, Fellow in Social Oncology, Dutch Cancer Foundation, The
Netherlands

Jennifer Hughes, M.R.C.P., M.R.C. Psych.
Senior Research Fellow, Department of Psychiatry, University of Southampton;
Honorary Consultant Psychiatrist, Royal South Hants Hospital, Southampton,
U.K.

Martin S. Lee, M.B., B.S., M.R.C. Psych.
Senior Registrar, Department of Psychiatry, Guy's Hospital, London, U.K.

S.J. Leinster, B.Sc., F.R.C.S. (Ed)
Senior Lecturer and Consultant Surgeon, Department of Surgery, University of
Liverpool, U.K.

Bernard S. Linn, M.D.
Professor of Surgery, University of Miami School of Medicine; Associate Chief
of Staff for Education, Veteran's Administration Medical Center, Miami,
U.S.A.

Margaret W. Linn, Ph.D.
Professor of Psychiatry, University of Miami School of Medicine; Director,
Social Science Research, Veteran's Administration Medical Center, Miami,
U.S.A.

Richard R. Love, M.D., M.S.
Associate Professor of Human Oncology, University of Wisconsin, Madison, U.S.A.

Martin G. Mott, B.Sc., M.B., F.R.C.P., D.C.H.
Senior Lecturer and Consultant Paediatrician, Department of Child Health, University of Bristol, U.K.

David R. Nerenz, Ph.D.
Chief, Great Lakes Regional Veteran's Administration Health Services Research and Development Program, Ann Arbor, U.S.A.

T.J. Priestman, M.D., F.R.C.P., F.R.C.R.
Consultant in Radiotherapy and Oncology, Dudley Road and Queen Elizabeth Hospitals, Birmingham, U.K.

J.F.A. Pruyn,
Social Psychologist, IVA, Institute for Social Scientific Research of the University of Tilburg, The Netherlands

Leslie R. Schover, Ph.D.
Assistant Professor of Urology (Psychology), Section of Sexual Rehabilitation, Department of Urology, M.D. Anderson Hospital, Houston, U.S.A.

Bryan A. Skinner,
Late of Grey Gables, Rue de Bocage, La Haule, St. Brelade, Jersey, Channel Islands, U.K.

Basil A. Stoll, F.R.C.R., F.F.R.
Honorary Consultant Physician to Oncology Departments, St. Thomas' Hospital and Royal Free Hospital, London, U.K.

H.W. Van den Borne,
Social Psychologist, IVA, Institute for Social Scientific Research of the University of Tilburg, The Netherlands

Maggie Watson, Ph.D.
Faith Courtauld Unit for Human Studies in Cancer, King's College, Hospital, London, U.K.

Avery D. Weisman, M.D.
Professor of Psychiatry, Massachusetts General Hospital and Harvard Medical School, Boston, U.S.A.

Elisabeth Whipp, M.A., F.R.C.R.
Consultant Radiotherapist and Oncologist, Bristol Royal Infirmary; Lecturer in Radiotherapy and Oncology, University of Bristol, U.K.

This book is
dedicated to the
memory of

BRYAN SKINNER

A tribute to his courage in the face of cancer and his constant hope that others
might benefit from his hard-won wisdom

Preface

The emotional pressures on cancer patients and their families are increasing and traditional supports are decreasing. This book attempts to provide a readable, authoritative and balanced review of the emotional pressures and coping methods of cancer patients, and the help currently available to them. The special problems of children and terminal patients with cancer, and the role of the family in coping, are also examined.

A balanced and critical assessment is made of defects in health organisation, training of personnel and attitudes to cancer patients in Western society. A similar assessment is made of the growing tendency to self help, mutual help and group activities for such patients. While each individual needs to select coping aids best suited to his or her own temperament, medical advisors need to make more time available for discussion of technical, emotional, social and sexual problems. The availability of a cancer-treating "team" makes this feasible.

Chapters were invited from physicians, psychiatrists, psychologists and sociologists expert in this field, and they have responded to the challenge of writing in non-technical language. This is so that readership can cross disciplinary boundaries and thus stimulate physicians, nurses, psychologists, sociologists, clergy and others, to satisfy some of the currently unmet needs of cancer patients. The reader may note a small amount of overlap between some chapters, permitted in order to maintain continuity and make each chapter complete in itself.

London, 1986   Basil A. Stoll

Contents

Introduction

AVERY D. WEISMAN

These are difficult times for practitioners and researchers in psychosocial oncology and the truly important questions are still with us: What can be done about problems that we don't understand as yet, and can scarcely formulate? How shall we differentiate between facts and traditional fictions?

There is still another question. Actual discoveries and encouraging developments have been accomplished over the past few decades, yet, it is not at all cynical to wonder what impact, if any, these discoveries have made upon cancer care, as it is generally understood. That cancer stress occurs is self-evident but what is really being done about it? There are ethical, scientific, and clinical dilemmas that surround cancer patients, cancer caregivers, and those bystanders who survive and suffer the depredations of a desperate disease in someone they love. Do we merely improvise, or seek out reliable information?

Every cancer patient has a unique contribution to make. Problems differ, yet certain general principles apply. Among these are distinct points of vulnerability that should alert clinicians to incipient difficulties. Moreover, these "pressure points" open up questions for inquiry, investigation, and research, if genuine progress is to be made. The authentic meaning of the so-called holistic approach depends on the blend of generality, specificity, and relevance to the unique case.

This book is not a mere reiteration of what has been said again and again in the mounting multitide of publications and symposia. It addresses a central question: How can we cope well enough with cancer stress, maintaining sufficient morale, with strong courage to face adversity – and still formulate pertinent questions that can be understood and applied wisely? But this central question is only the beginning. Specifics are needed, and these require enlightened concern, collaboration between specialties and disciplines, and, in the phrase now popular, transfer of technologies.

In simple terms, we need to share data, case material, adopt a comprehensible language, and encourage mutual referral, with minimal attention to the traditional hierarchies within medicine. Cancer care is far too important to be left to the physicians. After all, most truly original ideas come from outside the traditional establishment. Cancerology, as I prefer to dub this work of ours, needs all the new ideas, applications, and collaboration it can honestly get. There should be no cult of personality within the field. Essential though they are, pain control, home care, hospices, and enlightened economic policies do not exhaust the range of psychosocial oncology.

Too often, psychosocial research in this field leans on personality inventories and clinical rating scales, forgetting about or mistrusting direct personal observation and acumen. In the search for reproducible results, which are usually too general, even vapid, to mean anything, more subtle emotional predicaments and uncategorized varieties of distress are left unattended. Absorption with service can disregard general issues, just as clinical investigation can minimize the unique and suffering person who has cancer.

Therefore, the main prerequisites for coping with cancer in all its manifestations are familiarity with emotional pressure points, and respectful recognition of a wide range of coping strategies. The following distinct pressure points should be heeded:

Unexpected Resurgence of Unmitigated Pessimism

Most cancer patients tend to manage themselves rather well, from the time of initial diagnosis throughout the course, even to terminality. They cope inconspicuously, and their distress is not prominent enough to be noticed clinically. Others do well for a time, and then at various psychosocial phases, falter and regress. They voice concern about their plight, as if all further procedures will be in vain. While optimism can be deceptive, unmitigated pessimism is a noxious symptom.

Indifference to Social Supports

A little help goes a long way, but what, exactly, constitutes positive as contrasted with negative supportive efforts? Often, what is blithely intended to be supportive not only is not, but may undermine a precarious equilibrium. How any supportive intervention is interpreted depends on the readiness and mind-set of the patient. The so-called empathic window is often cloudy, and it is difficult to offer consistently positive support at all times. But when a cancer patient actively becomes numb and indifferent to everything done to help or sustain comfort and morale, then the submerged distress should be investigated, without further hesitation.

Repudiation of Available Help

This pressure point goes beyond numbness and indifference. Patients suddenly become irascible, bitter, and uncooperative. They are hard to take care of, and few caregivers are so forgiving and forbearing that they tolerate such "lack of appreciation." As a result, they show withdrawal and repudiation on their own, setting up a cycle of mutual misunderstanding that only deepens a rift.

Failure to Thrive

Who can tolerate persistent disappointment, frustration, and disfigurement of body and spirit, when, despite every effort and enterprise, deleterious symptoms and physical decline predominate? Looking in the mirror provides a moment of truth far more convincing than the reassuring words of compassionate caregivers. "How can I feel good, or believe I'm improving, when I can hardly walk and feel so rotten?"

Impersonalization

When the disease takes over completely, impersonalization becomes a fact, and the person becomes a mere case, a fragile vessel containing disseminated malignancy. This is a dire, desperate event of existential significance. To restore that patient's sense of self-esteem requires every therapeutic ingenuity.

Erosion of Autonomy

This is a nonspecific pressure point that is cumulative and progressive, without being marked by singular symptoms. Many patients who refrain from asking help are considered very cooperative. But upon closer attention, these patients passively submit to almost anything; they stop caring for themselves, as if nothing matters. They act helpless, and tolerate exceedingly uncomfortable situations, such as a full bladder, sleepless nights, or an impacted bowel. They behave as if no choice or option remains.

Demoralization

Few clinicians adequately differentiate between depression, which is a transient mood, and demoralization, which indicates a collapse of hope in one's ability to cope. Yet, morale and its maintenance is perhaps the key ingredient in separating those who will cope from those who will despair and deteriorate.

Poor Communication

Who is the first to recognize that communication between caregivers and cancer patient has broken down? Often enough, it is the observant, outside consultant who notices that whatever is said seems to be fragmentary and misunderstood. Words are given the opposite meaning from what is intended, and interventions meant to be encouraging are interpreted as somewhat hostile and uncaring. Clinicians who care also care about clear communication, and therefore are alert to what is said, understood, and recalled.

Emotional Extremes

Coping well is almost impossible when a patient is fixed at an emotional extreme, such as dejection, truculence, and anxiety. Excessive agitation of any sort impairs judgment; impaired judgment leads to cognitive distortion, and cognitive distortion may be the forerunner to confusion.

Denial in Excess

A little denial never hurt anyone; otherwise, most of us would be seriously damaged. To a degree, denial is somewhat useful for cancer patients, and their caregivers. Indeed, it is inevitable. But it is useful as a strategy only for a short time, under special circumstances, and is not to be encouraged in the long run. The purpose of denial is to transmogrify an important problem into an insignificant non-problem, which then does not need coping with. In excess, denial chases out other strategies, thereby increasing, not really relieving distress.

I did not intend to write an expository paper as part of this Introduction, but the importance of coping with cancer stress and its hazardous manifestations cannot be overemphasized, if we are to be truly conscientious about our vocation. Dr. Stoll has persuaded outstanding authorities to join with him im producing what should become the inspiration for a new forward surge in psychosocial oncology, a thrust in expert documentation that may provide the impetus for creative work into the next century, now so close at hand.

Suppose that by the time the 21st century comes around, an unlikely event shall have occurred. This event is the complete elucidation of the cancer problem. Not only would the neoplastic process be understood in its various forms, but treatment would be inexpensive, painless, available, asymptomatic, and certain. Only then might the problem of dealing with cancer stress also be eradicated, because stress would almost surely be minimal.

Meanwhile, cancer can drain the emotions as surely as it can deplete financial resources. How to take care of the multiple complications and ramifications of stress and distress is almost as essential as finding a better substitute for the relatively inadequate treatments of today. In our present state of knowledge, coping with cancer must combine hope with realism. Because complete cures are still virtually beyond the horizon, care and comfort deserve scrupulous study, coupled with pertinent research, stripped of all sentimentality, platitudes, and lugubrious metaphysics.

Patients who cope well enough tend to ask questions and insist upon sensible answers, not evasions. They share concern without being maudlin, and in response, are given reliable, up-to-date information, with free admission of ignorance, when needed. They also avoid stereotyping themselves, confronting problems that are practical and have a reasonable chance of being solved. If length of life cannot be extended, then the quality of life that remains becomes an uppermost consideration, so that an appropriate and acceptable death takes place.

Dr. Stoll's earlier books have prepared us for the fulfilment of these aims. He and his collaborators adopt a perspective that combines research data with long clinical experience. They avoid the easy nostrums of self-proclaimed experts, and respect the mystery that still envelops cancer, the malignant metaphor and agonizing reality of our age.

Readers should be aware that whatever is said and surmised about cancer patients may also be relevant for themselves. How mankind copes with cancer and its stresses can be a guide for coping with a host of other problems and maladies. Thus, regardless of our training, discipline, and disposition, we monitor problems, confront clearly, seek trustworthy guidance, undertake corrective actions – and then are ready to cope with the next problem at hand.

Avery D. Weisman, M.D.

PART ONE

IMPACT OF CANCER ON THE PATIENT

Chapter 1

Faith only belongs in Churches?

BASIL A. STOLL

This chapter title is derived from a remark which I heard recently from the Director of a well known Cancer Center in the USA. He said "faith only belongs in churches", implying that whether o not the patient had faith in his recovery was an irrelevancy to the doctor using modern powerful drugs to treat cancer. In fact, today's pressures on cancer patients are such as to demand every ounce of their faith if they are to cope with the physical and emotional stresses which are thrust upon them. This refers not only to religious faith but also to faith in their physicians and faith in their own ability to help themselves to recovery.

The past 25 years have seen cancer patients in Western countries subjected to much greater and more prolonged emotional strains than ever before. One major cause of stress is the increasing trend, supported by legal obligations, for doctors to disclose to cancer patients the full details of their diagnosis and their likely life expectancy. Following this, they are often offered a choice between alternative treatments and a list of all possible complications of the treatment which is selected.

The increased stress also reflects some of the marked social changes which have occurred in Western society in recent years. These include increasing distrust of experts, less religious faith, less family support and less personal rapport with the family doctor. All these factors make it harder for patients to make difficult decisions about treatment which will impair the quality of their lives. This applies especially in advanced cancer when decisions may have to be made regarding the major dilemma of Western medicine – whether life should be dragged on at all costs, irrespective of the quality.

In addition, there are the physical and emotional strains associated with the repeated, aggressive and prolonged cancer treatments which are commonly used today. While some patients are so hard hit by treatment that they may refuse to complete it, others become pathetically treatment- dependent, and begin to worry as the end of each treatment course approaches. These prolonged treatments are usually accompanied by repeated unconfortable monitoring investigations, which themselves contribute to the patient's anxiety. The persistent searching by the doctor may make the patient fearful that something vital may be overlooked and this often leads to constant anxiety about the results of the tests.

The purpose of this introductory chapter is to set out the major social, legal and medical changes in the past 25 years which have enormously increased the emotional strain on the cancer patient. It may help in understanding some current controversies in the emotional and psychological support of cancer patients. It may help to explain the head-on clash which we are seeing between orthodox and so called "alternative" unproven treatments, in which the confused cancer patient is the unfortunate victim.

Later chapters provide detailed discussion on how the cancer patient can be helped to cope with the stresses of the disease and the various treatments employed. This brief review emphasises the emotional pressures on the patient under the headings of;
- Anxiety is increasing
- Traditional supports are less
- Treatment is more aggressive
- Is faith a key factor in coping?

Anxiety is Increasing

A remarkable change in the medical climate came about in the United States between the years of 1961 and 1978; the proportion of patients who were frankly informed of their diagnosis of cancer rose from 10% to 98%. This change in medical attitudes is said to have resulted from changes in social opinions as to rights of patients to be informed (1). Equally, if not more important however, were the pressures from legal actions which forced doctors in the U.S.A. to practise defensive medicine - that is, to do what is legally safe, rather than what may be medically desirable in the circumstances.

Mass education has led to healthy distrust of experts and there is now considerable emphasis on the right of the individual to control his own living and dying. The patient now expects to be involved in all discussions and decisions affecting his treatment. It is however, unfortunate for his peace of mind that the cancer patient's expectations are often shattered by such discussions. He often discovers that many long standing dogmas have recently been rejected, and that there is considerable uncertainty as to the long-term efficacy of many accepted cancer treatments. He finds also that most decisions as to treatment in cancer involve a trade-off between inevitable side effects or mutilation, as against unguaranteed gains. Whereas previously, the physician made the decision on the patient's behalf, the patient and relatives are now presented with difficult choices and subsequently have to live with the results of the decision they take.

There is increasing opposition to paternalistic decisions by the physician, and a trend towards full disclosure and informed consent by the patient. It is now claimed

(2) that knowing the diagnosis (a) helps patients worry less and find greater resourcefulness while uncertainty "paralyses the individual's coping mechanism"; (b) helps patients put their affairs in order and avoids alienation from a family which knows more than the patient. Based on such assumptions, it is advocated that today's physician must learn to accept patients' emotional manifestations such as acute anxiety, depression, anger or hopelessness which follow full disclosure. He must learn to help patients and their families deal with the resulting problems (2).

Writers on the subject frequently support their arguments in favour of full disclosure by a report on the questioning of 256 advanced cancer patients in the U.S.A. (3). Among younger patients, about 90% said they wished to participate in management decisions and wanted all information about their disease, whether good or bad. (The figure was lower in older patients). But the study also showed that the patients who asked for most information were also the most optimistic ones. However bad the prospects which were revealed, they believed first, that something could be done to control their disease, and second that they personally would beat the odds.

Another commonly quoted report is on the questioning of 190 Canadian cancer patients with advanced cancer (4). Again 90% said that they wanted as much information as possible about their disease, and again 97% of all patients believed that they themselves would have their disease either cured or controlled by treatment. It is obvious from both reports that while most patients in North America may ask for all news both good and bad, given bad news they protect themselves from its impact by the conviction that they personally are going to beat the disease. If you were to try and convince them of the real odds against them it is likely that they would either ignore it or show hostility and depression (5).

Attitudes to full disclosure are quite different in Europe. In 1976, an enquiry among cancer patients in the U.K. showed that only about one in three wanted confirmation of a diagnosis of cancer, while only one in seven wished to be informed of the likely prognosis (6). Most patients merely wanted a progress report and reassurance at each visit. Another U.K. report on 200 patients with advanced lung cancer, showed that only about half the patients who were offered more information about their diagnosis, accepted the offer (7).

In the U.K. and in Europe generally, it is therefore customary for the doctor to be guided by the patient's questions, in deciding on how much information to give as to diagnosis and prognosis. What the patient is told depends on how much he already knows, how he has reacted to it and how much more he may wish to know with regard to his special fears (8). The ethical question for the European physician is not what information the patient is entitled to, but what information he believes is acceptable, and what the patient's real wishes and needs are. For the majority of patients in Europe this selective and compassionate variety of "paternalism" is clearly preferable to a confrontational "take it or leave it" attitude.

In recent years however, patient's rights to information about their disease and treatment have been stressed and this has been reinforced by legal obligations upon the doctor. Consent must of course be obtained before any treatment, but while this used to be tacitly assumed by the patient submitting to treatment, written consent is now required after detailed explanation of the nature and implications of the disease, and the possible complications of treatment (so-called "informed" consent). These changes have done away with much of the euphemisms, and bland reassurance of cancer patients which were common until recently in Europe. Informed consent is currently being obtained from the large number of patients now being enrolled in trials of new treatments.

A major problem for the cancer patient is that the term cancer is used broadly to cover 40 or 50 different types of tumour, each with very different characteristics. How many patients know that the proportion of tumours cured can vary from 1% to 99% according to the cancer type; that incurable cases can range from an indolent condition growing slowly over 30 years to a bushfire course over a few months? Almost universally, the diagnosis of "cancer" is emotionally charged and evokes the image of invalidism, incapacity and inevitable death, regardless of the real prognosis and available treatment.

The patient and family often ask how much time is left. Yet, any attempt to predict the course in the individual cancer patient can only be based on an overall statistic for each particular type of tumour. On this may be superimposed the guess of the doctor as to the individual's prognosis, at a similar level to that of a punter guessing which horse will win a race. This being so, it is clear that any physician who commits himself to a specific prognosis when the patient first presents, shows himself ignorant of the gross variation in cancer behaviour between individuals. There is obviously no place for the words "never" or "always" when talking of the prognosis of cancer.

The legal requirement now common in the U.S.A., which confronts the patient with a list of all known complications of a treatment, is still regarded as counterproductive in Europe and the U.K. On the basis that a full list of every rare complication might deter a patient from a treatment which the doctor considers in the patient's interest, he tells the patient only of the serious and reasonably probable risks of treatment. He thus provides advice to guide a patient through an inevitably highly complex trade-off of advantages against drawbacks. Nevertheless, demands for totally complete information are increasing from patient pressure groups even in Europe and the U.K. and are being backed by medicolegal action. Do all patients really want to know every possible complication of every treatment they receive?

Traditional Supports are Less

Coping with a diagnosis of cancer requires considerable courage from the patient and constant support from the family. However, family support is less than it used to be, and many older patients live alone with their fears. It is widely agreed that emotional stress is more common among cancer patients either with little family support or poor emotional resources. Most people need to be able to talk through their anxieties with others, in the same way as do individuals after bereavement, and also to give vent to tears, anger or other emotions. Western society does not encourage this, at least not in public.

The diagnosis of cancer can place a severe strain on family relationships. It was often customary to tell the family the prognosis, but to withhold it from the patient at the family's request: it is now more common to give the patient and family the information at the same time, thus bringing them together and avoiding a barrier between the patient and the relatives. But this may create its own problems. Fear that the disease is in the family ("grandfather died of cancer of the prostate and now father has lung cancer"), or that the disease may be infectious (a misconception stimulated by reports in the media about the relationship between viruses and cancer). The patient may thus see himself as unclean, a danger to others and shunned by those around.

In the public mind, the word cancer represents a death sentence and the vast majority of people in modern Western society have not come to terms with death. In bygone days, old people died at home surrounded by relatives, young and old, whereas now the majority die in hospitals, and children are not encouraged to attend either funerals or cemeteries. Death is swept under the carpet. One of the first needs of cancer patients therefore, is to come to terms with mortality, and in fact a considerable proportion become more religious after learning the diagnosis, particularly among younger patients (3).

Publicity in the popular media provides lay education but at the same time provokes considerable fear of cancer because of the more sensational aspects which tend to be reported. News items usually refer to notabilities dying of cancer, but rarely of those pursuing a normal life after succesful treatment (unless of course, that treatment has been attributed to unorthodox medicine). In addition, the media repeatedly publicise major "breakthroughs" in medicine, so that cancer patients and relatives may develop unrealistic expectations which cannot be satisfied.

Medical care has changed as Western society has changed. Earlier in the century, when the patient faced serious illness, the family doctor helped to spare the patient and family from difficult decisions and subsequent regret and recrimination. Where once such decisions might be taken without question by a figure of authority, our "high-tech", materialist Western society has destroyed a large part of this relationship. This is evident particularly in North America.

The new values encourage the belief that health and longevity are available somewhere, but that you have to shop around to find them. In a generally irreligious society, death is no longer regarded as the friend of the very sick and aged, but rather as the ultimate enemy who must be repeatedly beaten off whatever the cost. Should a doctor question the artificial prolongation of a life that is not truly living, many would be outraged.

Treatment is more Aggressive

Because there has been little improvement in the cure rates for the majority of common cancers in the last 30 years, there is a trend to increasingly aggressive treatment in the hope of prolonging life. In former years, the patient with early cancer received the selected primary treatment by surgery or radiotherapy. He then reported back at long intervals, or earlier if suspicious symptoms suggested possible recurrence of the disease. Currently, however, many cancer patients are being treated continuously for years by new agents, in the hope of delaying recurrence. This applies both in early and advanced cancer.

Participation in such trials requires the informed consent of the patient, in the course of which the patient is made aware that the degree of benefit from treatment is uncertain. Having committed himself to such a trial, it is then common for the patient to learn from the media or his friends of other "promising" treatments which have been discovered. All this makes it hard for the patient to make a decision and live with the results, especially with the burden of information about his disease which the patient must receive in order to participate in the trial. The emotional stress is considerable.

Add to this the unpleasant side effects of most types of chemotherapy and the burden of repeated visits to the hospital for treatment and investigation. At the very least, it postpones the patient's enjoyment of normal life until the long course is finished, and involves a constant state of anxiety as to how the disease is progressing. The hope of prolonging life is the bait. If successful, such treatment may indeed postpone recurrence, but if it finally occurs, the whole cycle of treatment and investigation has to be endured once more.

Oncologists have a tendency to underestimate the unpleasant side effects of their treatment because of various inadequacies in the doctor/patient relationship (9). Doctors who are not involved in research trials are in a dilemma over treatments where only a few patients will benefit while all have to undergo repeated visits to the hospital, repeated investigations and the side effects of treatment. How do you balance so much stress against an uncertain chance of control? Obviously the patient must make such a choice, but is it any wonder that he is highly anxious?

Unfortunately, the technological improvement in medical practice has eroded the traditional doctor/patient relationship. Responsibility for the cancer patient rarely belongs to one doctor but is now shared by a team, with the surgeon, radiation therapist and specialist medical oncologist contributing at different stages of the disease. Although such a group provides greater expertise and greater information for the patient, it does not necessarily provide a greater degree of emotional support. In fact, discussion of psychosocial problems tends to suffer as scientific investigations multiply, and few doctors are inclined to probe for emotional problems. A cancer patient's widow graphically describes these problems in the following comment on her husband's medical care (10):

"Two major weaknesses emerged. When it was finally admitted that drugs or technology could do nothing more, the nurses continued to provide care and attention; the doctors disappeared with the drips, antibiotics and blood. Perhaps their training has not taught them how to meet failure; perhaps they need to protect themselves; perhaps they have nothing to give if technology fails. The second weakness was the result of specialisation.... the patient may come under several specialties all concerned with a particular part of the body and no one doctor appears to be responsible for the whole patient".

Is Faith a Key Factor in Coping?

How then does today's cancer patient cope with the increased confrontations, the decreased support and the increased stresses of modern treatment?

The result of legal, social and medical pressures is that the vast majority of patients are being confronted by their diagnosis of cancer. Although the term is a loose one, it is interpreted by the patient as a likely death sentence, irrespective of what is added afterwards by way of explanation. In fact, he may even fail to absorb the explanation in the shock of the word "cancer".

Individual patients react differently, according to their temperament and emotional resources. Nevertheless, shock and denial which are the normal reaction to apparent sentence of death, are probably the initial predominant emotions in most cases. The subsequent coping strategy chosen by the patient (dependency on others, religious faith, positive action, optimism or nonacceptance of the seriousness of the disease) depends mainly on his habitual method of coping with severe stress. While some patients try to solve their problems in a rational way, others behave emotionally.

The aim of the clinician should be to recognise the patient's predominant coping method at different times in the course of the disease. But having recognised it, doctors' opinions differ as to management. Some believe that unrealistic coping behaviour, such as denial or belief in unproven practices, should be discouraged in favour of a realistic appraisal of the situation. Others believe that the patient's own chosen strategy should be encouraged and that it is wrong to impose the clinician's norms of coping behaviour or scientific attitude on a patient.

Coping with an immediate threat to life is a very basic instinct. In animals it involves physical activity (fight or flight) as an alternative to complete surrender to fear. In the case of man, coping may involve an additional dimension – faith or hope that something will happen to remove the threat. Whether the coping strategy of the cancer patient is going to be active or passive, there must be underlying faith in recovery, hope and will-to-live: without this, the patient would fall into a state of utter fear, helplessness and depression.

How does the cancer patient maintain this faith over a prolonged period? Every individual establishes his or her own distinctive method involving a mixture of selection or suppression of items, confrontation or avoidance of facts, acceptance or denial of the threat (11).

People vary in their concept as to how far they control their own lives – psychologically this is called their concept of "locus of control". Cancer patients with a more internal locus of control feel more in charge of their own life and illness, so that they will tend to deny that the condition is as serious as might appear, or else they have faith that they are strong enough to beat it. To deny the feeling of helplessness caused by the diagnosis, they may take certain positive steps (e.g. changes in diet or habits) to assert their own control over their health. On the other hand, those with a more external locus of control prefer to put their faith in outside agencies to help them to recovery. They commonly put their trust in prayer, family or medical attendants.

Thus, there are two major stereotypes to which the vast majority of Western patients tend to conform:

1. The confident and more aggressive patient. He asks the clinician for considerable information, but mainly in the hope of finding reassurance. He seeks every orthodox treatment available, and information about unorthodox treatments in addition. He refuses to accept bad news or its implications, or else he believes that he can beat the odds against him. He would break down or become very angry if forced to accept the truth of a serious prognosis. This attitude is the one most commonly seen among patients in the U.S.A.

2. The stoic and more philosophic patient. He accepts the diagnosis but has confidence in his medical advisors, and knows that all that can be done will be done. He often becomes more religious and more believing. He does not ask many questions but prefers as far as possible, to carry on his previous life style accepting each day as it comes. This attitude is the one most commonly seen among patients in the U.K. and Europe.

It is clear from the above that there is, in general, a difference between the attitudes of American and European cancer patients to their disease, and it reflects their different attitudes to health problems overall. The American patient tends to seek more information but takes a positive attitude to his illness. He intends to keep going and believes he can help his body fight the disease and get well. This attitude may apply less as patients become increasingly ill because their belief in being able to control their own destiny has to give way to increasing dependence on the physician (3). The European patient's attitude is more to avoid unnecessary information, maintain confidence in his medical advisors and expect them to provide the care necessary to keep him going. This basic difference in attitude to all health matters is well known, and is taken into account by most advertising agencies when they pubilcise the same sell health products both in the U.S.A. and in Europe.

We noted earlier that in the U.S.A. it is generally advocated that all cancer patients should have full disclosure of all information about their disease, on the basis that helping patients fully face up to their problem makes them better able to cope emotionally (12). It is said that the provision of full information to cancer patients does not create depression, but actually assists many of them to maintain hopeful attitudes; that confirmation of the diagnosis ends a state of uncertainty which may be worse than knowing the facts (3). Yet in the U.K., a report suggests that 70% of patients who suspected that they had malignant disease did not want to know for certain. As long as they were uncertain, they found it easier to maintain hope (6).

The American tendency to treat the diagnosis of cancer as an emotional hurdle or crisis which the patient needs to confront and then overcome, is questioned not only in Europe but also by some American authorities (13). Cancer is frequently a chronic disease prolonged over a period of many years during which the patient goes about his or her normal activities. As used in the title of this book, the term "coping" is intended to mean adjustment to a chronic problem rather than to overcoming an acute crisis.

It is time for clinicians treating cancer to seriously question the proposition that by making patients confront their cancer as a crisis situation, we are facilitating positive coping attitudes and acceptance. While in the general problems of life, there is no doubt that positive coping is improved as a result of directly confronting a problem, this has not been proved for cancer (14). Let us not make a virtue out of necessity. Confrontation with the problems of cancer diagnosis and treatment has arisen as a result of social and legalistic pressures. Some would justify it on the same basis that terminal patients are presently encouraged to accept their dying state, but, as is made clear in the previous paragraph, the situations are not comparable.

A few cancer patients can accept blunt talk about a bad prognosis, but most patients suffer a greater or lesser degree of anxiety or depression because the impact of what they have been told is intolerable (14,15). Weisman (16) defines coping with cancer as learning to tolerate something that was previously intolerable and advises that the patient should learn to confront his problem as soon as possible. On the other hand, Silberfarb (13) believes that succesful coping by the cancer patient may require postponing acceptance of the condition. But whichever course is adopted, the patient's faith in recovery is the key to successful coping, and in some patients this may involve refusal to accept the seriousness of the disease.

If cancer is a chronic disease, a degree of denial is not only permissible but it should actually be encouraged for the purpose of maintaining faith and hope in recovery. It is common for cancer patients to refuse to accept fully what they prefer not to face, although the degree of denial may vary from time to time. For example, in a group of 100 cancer patients in the U.S.A. who were told the diagnosis at the time of initial treatment, almost half the men (although less of the women) subsequently denied that they knew their diagnosis, and an even higher proportion denied the seriousness of their condition (17). The North American studies referred to earlier, whose paradoxical findings were that patients who asked for most information were also the most optimistic (3) (4), confirms a high capacity for denial in the majority of cancer patients ("even if only a few survive, I will be amongst them").

A cancer patient has expressed this feeling very clearly "I am very much against the use of statements such as 'you have cancer' without some understanding of how the patient will interpret it. To many, cancer means terminal illness and a protracted painful death with no hope of escaping either the disease or its treatment. I therefore see it as a healthy sign when patients refuse to accept fully that they have cancer. These patients need healthy imaginings to maintain their morale and fight off the depressing image of a helpless victim" (18).

The last few years have seen considerable support for the healthy use of denial (non acceptance of the seriousness of the disease) by cancer patients. A recent report suggests that making a patient confront the full implications of the diagnosis of breast cancer makes coping more difficult in the short term (15). There is evidence that in the long term also, denial of the seriousness of the disease can help patients to cope, even when tumour recurrence has occurred (19).

There are also reports that cancer patients who avoid facing their illness as a crisis by using denial or optimism, not only enjoy a greater freedom from anxiety but also survive longer than those who show passive acceptance of their condition (20). If a positive and optimistic attitude may prolong survival, is it helpful to force the patient into a confrontation crisis which will undermine such optimism?

In order to strengthen their belief in their own ability to help themselves, many patients seek active methods of self help in addition to the orthodox treatment which they may be receiving. Even a placebo may help to increase the patient's faith in himself, so that such practices should not be denigrated. In addition, many of the commonly used self help practices help also to reduce nervous tension. Among a group of 78 breast cancer patients in the U.S.A., about two thirds expressed their faith that they themselves could exert control over the progress of their cancers (19). To reinforce their faith, many had taken active steps in self help by diet, change in habits or meditation. These were claimed to have resulted in better emotional adjustment.

Patients may have a variety of motives for pursuing self help – a desire to explore every possible avenue, expectations which scientific medicine cannot satisfy, or failure of the physician to communicate in a compassionate manner. Yet many orthodox clinicians discourage the patient in the quest for self help on the basisthat unproven treatment is by definition of no value to the patient. What values are we referring to?

Faith is a word rarely used in orthodox medical writing, mainly because it does not sit comfortably with the scientific, technological training of modern doctors. It is rarely mentioned in the clinical or psychological literature because it is not measurable. Yet, Sir William Osler who set the scientific foundations of modern medicine, said that "faith was the doctor's most precious asset - the one great moving force which we can neither weigh in the balance nor test in the crucible". It is the failure of orthodox medicine to harness this key force (an example being the opening quote of this chapter) which has allowed practitioners of alternative medicine to attract so many patients with cancer.

Conclusion

Cancer patients in the Western world are presently subject to much greater and more prolonged strains than ever they were in the past. Not only is medical treatment more aggressive and social support less effective, but in addition, legal and social changes have led to the vast majority of patients being confronted with "total" information about the details of their disease and possible life expectancy. This is claimed by some to facilitate positive coping attitudes and acceptance in cancer patients but such a claim has not been proved.

Each patient reacts differently to the impact of the diagnosis, and whereas some patients are anxious to do something active themselves, some are happy to let others help them to recovery. Patients should be encouraged in whatever steps they select to bolster their coping ability - dependency on others, religious faith, positive action or optimism. Refusal to accept the seriousness of the disease should not be discouraged.

The key factors to succesful coping in all patients are their faith, hope and will-to-live. Faith in recovery not only improves quality of life in all patients, it may also prolong life in some patients. The doctor who treats the patient's will-to-live as an irrelevance is guilty not only of arrogance but also of ignorance. Faith in recovery is an essential part of coping with cancer, even if, in our present state of knowledge, we are unable to measure it.

References

1. Novack, D.H., Plumer, R., Smith, R.L., Ochitill, H., Morrow, G.R., Bennett, J.M. (1979) Changes in physicians' attitudes toward telling the patient. Journal American Medical Association, 241,897–900.
2. Steinert, Y. (1985) What to tell cancer patients. Union International Contra Cancer, Newsletter, 3,11–12.
3. Cassileth, B.R., Zupkis, R.V., Sutton-Smith, K., March, V. (1980) Information and participation preferences among cancer patients. Annals of Internal Medicine, 92,832–836.
4. Eidinger, R.N., Schapira, D.V. (1984) Cancer patients' insights into their treatment, prognosis and unconventional therapies. Cancer, 53,2736–2740.
5. Muss, H.B., White, D.R., Michielutte, R., Richards, F., Cooper, M.R., Williams, S., Stuart, J.J., Spurr, C.L. (1979) Written informed consent in patients with breast cancer. Cancer, 43,1549–1556.
6. McIntosh, J. (1976) Patient's awareness and desire for information about diagnosed but undisclosed malignant disease. Lancet, 2,300–303.
7. Spencer-Jones, J. (1981) Telling the right patient. British Medical Journal, 283,291–292.
8. Calnan, J. (1983) Talking with patients. Heinemann Medical, London, p.12.
9. Parliament, M.B., Danjoux, C.E., Clayton, T. (1985) Is cancer treatment toxicity accurately reported? International Journal Radiation Oncology, 11,6033–608.

20

10. Anonymous (1983) Cancer; the relative's view. Lancet, 2,1188–1189.
11. Weisman, A. (1976) Coping behavior and suicide in cancer. In Cancer - the Behavioral Dimension (Eds. J.W. Cullen, B.H. Fox, R.N. Ison) Raven Press, New York, 331–341.
12. Ferlic, M., Goldman, A., Kennedy, B.J. (1979) Group counselling in adult patients with advanced cancer. Cancer, 43,760–766.
13. Silberfarb, P.M. (1982) Research in adaptation to illness and psychosocial intervention. Cancer, 50 (Suppl), 1921–1924.
14. Maguire, P. (1982) Psychological and social consequences of cancer. In Recent Advances in Clinical Oncology (Eds. C. Williams and M. Whitehouse) Churchill Livingstone, Edinburgh, 375–384.
15. Watson, M., Greer, S., Blake, S., Shrapnell, K. (1984) Reaction to a diagnosis of breast cancer. Cancer, 53,2008–2012.
16. Weisman, A. (1984) The Coping Capacity. Human Sciences Press, New York, p.31.
17. Leigh, H., Ungerer, J., Percarpio, B. (1980) Denial and helplessness in cancer patients undergoing radiation therapy. Cancer, 45,3086–3089.
18. Fiore, N. (1979) Fighting cancer - one patient's perspective. New England Journal Medicine, 284,289–291
19. Taylor, S. (1983) Adjustment to threatening events. American Psychologist November, 1983, 1161–1173.
20. Stoll, B.A. (1979) Mind and Cancer Prognosis. John Wiley, Chichester, p.183.

Chapter 2

Impact of Diagnosis on the Patient

T.J. PRIESTMAN

Doctors' attitudes to informing patients of their diagnosis have changed over the last 25 years (see Chapter 1) and more people are today aware that they have cancer (1, 2). The few reports on the impact of this increased awareness on patients are of two types. The first comes from experienced physicians, tends to be anecdotal and offers virtually no quantitative data. The second comes from psychologists and psychiatrists, is based on relatively small and precisely defined groups which provide quantitative data, but may rely on methods too complex or too obscure to be readily reproduced. In this chapter, three separate questions will be considered: what is the response of the individual to the diagnosis, what determines this response, and which responses are beneficial?

What is the Response to the Diagnosis?

Revelation of the diagnosis of cancer is inevitably traumatic and one recent survey in Scotland (3) has shown that almost 40 per cent of patients with lymphoma suffered significant psychiatric problems (predominantly anxiety or depression) following confirmation of the diagnosis. Senescu (4) has categorised the emotional problems which might develop, based on certain fundamental reaction of man to disease:

The dependency response: complex, prolonged investigation and treatment tend to make a patient dependent on the medical services. This may provoke two extremes of response – either a complete loss of initiative and responsibility so that the patient comes to rely totally on the medical and support services for all his needs, or else a patient who struggles to retain total independence because he sees his need for reliance on others as humiliating and threatening.

Loss of self-esteem: the feeling that having cancer is a major physical imperfection and that one is irreparably damaged as a result.

Anger: as an anticipatory response to actual or threatened pain or damage. This may be non-specific and directed against fate or "the unfairness of it all" or focussed on a particular aspect of the disease or treatment, or sometimes on an individual.

Guilt: this may exist in addition to other responses and may have many sources. These include a belief that the cancer is a punishment for some previous misdemeanour, a feeling of guilt for envying healthy friends and relatives or guilt at the distress and inconvenience one is causing the family.

Loss of gratification: the patient can no longer enjoy previous pleasures and withdraws into a state of total lack of interest in outside stimuli.

In a survey (quoted in (5)), 53 physicians caring for cancer patients were asked to identify the frequency of various psychosocial problems in cancer patients, and the percentages noted below indicate the proportion of doctors who replied 'almost always' to each category. It should be noted that financial problems are high up on the list, and a study has shown the very severe financial hardship (with consequent emotional disruption for family members) that can result from the presence of cancer in a child (6).

Feelings of depression or hopelessness 36%

Fears or preoccupation 34%

Financial problems 32%

Occupational difficulties 23%

Feelings of helplessness or loss of control 17%

Feelings of loneliness or isolation 17%

Disruption of family role 15%

Loss of self-esteem 13%

Problems in sexual activity 11%

Feelings of anger 9%

Disinterest in social activity 9%

Fear of disfigurement 8%

The immediate psychological response to diagnosis has been defined in a study of women in the U.K. with carcinoma of the breast (7). Sixty-nine women were assessed before mastectomy and again three months after surgery, by structured interviews and a battery of psychological tests. Two major conclusions emerged: the first was that psychological responses to breast cancer could be defined into four mutually exclusive categories; the second was that they could be correlated with length of survival. The categories were:

- Stoic acceptance (56% patients): Initial distress followed by acknowledgement of the diagnosis and a determination to carry on normal life, seeking no further information about their illness and ignoring its presence as far as possible.

- Denial (17% patients): No apparent emotional distress but active rejection of any knowledge of the diagnosis or evidence of their disease.

- Fighting spirit (17% patients): No apparent emotional distress but adoption of an optimistic attitude, expression of a will to do everything possible to beat the disease and a desire for more information about it.

- Helplessness/hopelessness (10% patients): Obviously distressed, totally overwhelmed by the disease, viewing themselves as gravely ill and constantly preoccupied by cancer and fear of impending death.

TABLE 1 Survival in breath cahier patents in relation to their psychologual response to dotease (8).

| | Initially | Number alive | |
		At 5 years	At 10 years
Denial/fighting spirit	20	18	12
Stoic/hopelessness	37	23*	9**

*p<0.025 **p<0.01

The survival data showed that attitudes of denial or fighting spirit correlated with better five and ten-year (8) survival figures than did stoic acceptance or hopelessness (Table 1). However, this study examined only a relatively small number of patients and a larger, confirmatory study is currently in progress. The study was restricted to women with carcinoma of the breast and although one may suspect similar psychological responses in patients with other tumours, it is important for the same methods to be applied in other cancers to see if these results have a more general relevance.

A great deal has been written about the psychological impact of breast cancer, and the impact of mastectomy is perhaps the best documented aspect of all. The incidence of psychological morbidity in such patients is well-established (9), but it is important to distinguish how far this is due to the trauma of mastectomy (see Chapter 3) and how far to the impact of the diagnosis. The emotional sequence in such cases is said to involve initial shock followed by disbelief, anxiety, anger, guilt and depression, and a subsequent period of readjustment during which these feelings ebb and flow until equilibrium is established or adjustment fails. Such failure was reflected by depression sufficiently severe to merit psychiatric intervention in 15–25% of women, and sexual problems in about 30% (9).

What Determines the Response?

The factors which determine the nature of a person's response to the diagnosis of cancer will vary with the individual but the majority fall under four headings: the disease and its treatment, the patient's personality: the patient's inter-personal relationships and the quality of relationships with nursing and medical staff.

The Disease and its Treatment

The problems associated with treatment are dealt with in more detail in other chapters, but fear engendered by the diagnosis needs emphasis. Fear is a major component in determining the response to any illness, and cancer is feared more than other diseases. The following are some of the reasons given for such fear among the public (10):

(a) A widespread belief that cancer is uniformly fatal, and that when death does occur, it is wretched and invariably painful. Many also believe that before cancer kills it mutilates.

(b) For many, cancer is still a uniquely unclean disease evoking feelings of contamination and disgust. It is regarded as a destruction from within, and represents the body destroying itself in a particularly frightening way. There is also a widespread belief that cancer is contagious

(c) The behaviour of cancer is unpredictable and even after apparent cure it may return. In addition, treatment is uniformly dreaded and the side-effects of therapy are often perceived as worse than the disease.

(d) The disease is arbitrary in whom it attacks, it is unjust and unfair in this random choice of victims, and this very randomness imputes guilt; there must be something the patient has done to deserve the condition.

Most of these beliefs are either untrue or gross misconceptions, yet undoubtedly they exist. There are few reports on how prevalent these views are, but one recent Scottish survey of knowledge on various aspects of breast cancer found strong correlations with age and social class (presumably equating with level of formal education). Within each social group, women between 30 and 49 years were significantly more knowledgeable about the disease ($p < 0.001$) than those older or younger, and levels of ignorance increased significantly with declining social class(11).

The dominant fears or concerns of individual patients probably vary with different cancers. While the major concern of most cancerpatients focusses on fears of recurrence, in the case of breast cancer concern over mutilation and sexuality seems to predominate, at least at the time of diagnosis.

The presence of "irrational" fears probably explains an observation which seems paradoxical: the level of distress induced by the diagnosis is as high in those with early, potentially curable disease, as in those with incurable cancer (12). Thus, merely revealing the diagnosis calls up numerous fears and misconceptions for which a bland reassurance that "the condition is curable" may be inadequate.

Personality of the Patient and Interpersonal Relationship

The relationship of coping to the prior personality of cancer patients and their social support is discussed in chapter 12. It has been shown that high neuroticism scores (as measured by the Eysenck personality inventory) are related to increased evidence of stress on learning the diagnosis in lymphoma patients (3), increased perception of pain in women with advanced carcinoma of the cervix (13) and a greater likelihood of failure to adjust to mastectomy (9).

A recent survey in patients with breast cancer, examined the change in personal relationships experienced by women following their diagnosis (10). Over 70% of the patients felt they were treated differently after people knew they had cancer, and of these, more than half found they were avoided or feared. Over 70% felt misunderstood, with inappropriate support or attitudes from family and friends heightening their sense of isolation. Only half the patients assessed the support they received as adequate to fill their needs, and only 40% reported that they had gained adequate support from either their husbands, family or friends. Furthermore, the level of support declined with increasing stage of disease.

Cancer still carries a social stigma often leading to isolation of the patient, as shown by the results of a questionnaire to 100 healthy individuals. Of these, 61 per cent said they might avoid contact with a friend who had cancer, yet paradoxically, if they had cancer only 15% anticipated that their own social contacts might diminish (10).

The Relationship with Nursing and Medical Staff

The interaction between patient and doctor is of major importance (see chapter 18) and one aspect of the relationship that has been examined in detail is the provision of information by the doctor and its impact on the patient (14). While most doctors in the U.K. would feel that honesty is desirable, they would not wish to be explicit with every patient. They prefer to "adapt to the patient's personality and background and to what seems to be going on in his mind" (15). Such a flexible policy also satisfies those who believe that the information needs of patients vary at different times during their illness (9,15).

That some patients may not wish to be fully informed was the conclusion from a Scottish study of patients with diagnosed but undisclosed malignancy (16). Of 74 patients, 18 knew they had cancer and 47 suspected the diagnosis. Of those who suspected, 69% did not want to know for certain, and overall only 14% of patients actually wanted information on their prognosis. In the U.S.A., enquiry as to which cancer patients are most likely to seek defenitive information from their clinicians found that younger and better educated people consistently desired more details than older and poorer educated individuals, and that the need was greatest at the time of initial diagnosis but declined thereafter (17). In the over 60's age group, 20 per cent indicated that they wanted only "minimal or good" information.

A proportion of patients are bound to be dissatisfied with the amount of information they receive. It has been shown that patient characteristics which predispose to such complaints are high levels of neuroticism, an initial perception of good health and apparent lack of concern at the diagnosis (3). The latter two points are interpreted as suggesting that these patients are less prepared for the emotional trauma of the diagnosis, and that their complaints about information levels reflect a generally more difficult adjustment to their cancer.

Which Responses are Beneficial?

We may classify response to the diagnosis of cancer under four patterns but more than one response may be apparent at the same time or different responses may appear sequentially. The patterns shown by patients may be:
- Therapeutic adaptation: Realistically appraising their symptoms, seeking medical advice, and co-operating with treatment in such a way as to maximise their chances of recovery or their adjustment to the disability caused by the cancer (18).
- Denial: Minimising, ignoring or rejecting the disease and its consequences.
- Hopelessness: Incorporating feelings of depression, guilt and anxiety.
- Anger: Varying degrees of hostility directed towards the disease itself or towards individuals, often compounded by feelings of unfairness and frustration.

Therapeutic adaptation is clearly desirable while hopelessness and anger are equally clearly maladaptive responses. The value of denial is hard to classify (see chapter 1) but the available evidence suggests that it is often an effective coping mechanism and does not appear to adversely affect survival (7).

On the other hand, negative feelings or attitudes which encourage maladaptive responses include:
- Uncertainty: This may refer to the course of the disease, the side-effects of treatment, the degree of disability that might be encountered, the complications of the illness or the ultimate prognosis.
- Loss of control: Feelings of powerlessness in the face of such a major illness and the usually complex and demanding therapy.
- Inability to identify any one person responsible for management: Patients are confused when multiple disciplines are involved in their therapy and there is no one individual to whom they can relate for advice, information and support.
- Loss of self-esteem: Feeling that having the disease makes them a damaged or second-rate person.
- Loss of gratification: Feeling that all the pleasure has gone out of life and there is nothing worth doing any more.
- Alienation and isolation: Feeling deserted by friends or family or socially excluded because of their cancer, and unable to meet naturally with other people because of the stigma of malignancy.

Conclusion

The chapter has identified consistent patterns of reaction to the diagnosis of cancer and some of the major influences on the responses observed. It is essential for clinicians to be aware of the emotional problems that the patient may encounter, so that they can be identified at an early stage of their development and appropriate steps taken to correct them.

References

1. Novack, D,H., Freireich, E.J., Vaisrub,S. (1979) Changes in the physician's attitude towards telling the cancer patient. Journal of the American Medical Association, 241, 897–900.
2. Anonymous (1980) In cancer, honesty is here to stay. Lancet, ii, 2445.
3. Lloyd G.G., Parker, A.C., Ludlam C.A., McGuire R.J. (1984) Emotional impact of diagnosis and early treatment of lymphomas. Journal of Psychosomatic Research, 28, 1577–162.
4. Senescu R.A. (1964) The development of emotional complications in the patient with cancer. Journal of Chronic Disease, 16, 813–832.
5. Luce J,K. (1979) Selecting patients for supportive therapy. In, Mind & Cancer Prognosis. (Ed. B. A. Stoll) John Wiley, Chichester. pp 127–137.
6. Bodkin C.M., Piggott, T.J., Mann J.R. (1982) Financial burden of childhood cancer. British Medical Journal, 284, 1542-1544.
7. Greer, S., Morris, T., Pettingale, K.W. (1979) Psychological response to breast cancer: effect on outcome. Lancet, ii, 785–787.
8. Pettingale, K.W. (1984) Coping and cancer prognosis. Journal of Psychosomatic Research, 28, 363–364.
9. Morris, T. (1983) Psychosocial aspects of breast cancer: a review. European Journal of Cancer and Clinical Oncology, 19, 1725–1733.
10. Peters-Golden, H. (1982) Breast cancer: varied perceptions of social support in the illness experience. Social Science & Medicine, 16, 483–491.
11. Roberts, M.M., French, K., Duffy, J. (1984) Breast cancer and breast self-examination: what do Scottish women know? Social Science & Medicine, 18, 791–797.
12. Gotay,, C.G. (1984) The experience of cancer during early and advanced stages: the views of patients and their mates. Social Science & Medicine, 18, 605–613.
13. Bond, M.R. (1971) The relation of pain to the Eysenck personality inventory, Cornell medical index and Whiteley index of hypochondriasis. British Journal of Psychiatry. 119, 671–678.
14. Aitken-Swan, J., Easson, E.C. (1959) Reactions of cancer patients on being told their diagnosis. Lancet, i. 779–783.
15. Brewin, T.B. (1977) The cancer patient: communication and morale. British Medical Journal, iv, 1623–1627.
16. McIntosh, J. (1976) Patients awareness and desire for information about diagnosed but undisclosed malignant disease. Lancet, ii, 300–303.
17. Cassileth, B.R., Zupkis, R.V., Sutton-Smith,K., March, V. (1980) Information and participation preferences among cancer patients. Annals of Internal Medicine, 92, 832–836.
18. Lloyd, G.C. (1979) Psychological stress and coping mechanisms in patients with cancer. In, Mind and Cancer Prognosis. (Ed B. A. Stoll) John Wiley, Chichester, pp 47–59.

TABLE 1. Survival in breast cancer patents in relation to their psychologual response to disease (8).

	Initially	Number alive At 5 years	At 10 years
Denial/fighting spirit	20	18	12
Stoic/hopelessness	37	23*	9**

*p < 0.025 **p < 0.01

Chapter 3

Coping with Cancer Surgery

S.J. LEINSTER

Doctors and other professionals can easily underestimate the anxiety engendered in a patient by the prospect of an operation. What to the professional may be routine, is often a once in a lifetime experience for the patient dying in an alien environment away from the support of family and friends. Usually he has two main areas of concern: the first is the degree of pain and discomfort he might have to suffer and the second is fear of the outcome.

Patients' unfamiliarity with surgical procedures may result in fantasies as to possible outcomes and in particular, they are afraid of the experience of loss of consciousness and the possibility of dying. When nursing staff caring for such patients were questioned, they tended to under-estimate the patients' concern about pain and discomfort, although their estimate of the level of fear was more accurate. They believed that they took active steps to reduce the patients' fear but the latter often did not recognise these interventions as such, thinking that the nurses were just "being friendly" (1).

In addition to the usual problems associated with surgery, patients with cancer have more long-term psychological distress including marked feelings of helplessness which can proceed to depression (2). In a comparison between cancer patients, general surgery patients and other patients, the cancer patients and surgery patients had more psychological distress than did other patients, while the cancer patients reported more marked feeling of helplessness than the non-cancer surgical patients, and also more prolonged psychological distress (3).

For the patient facing cancer, four main areas of concern exist:
- The fact of having cancer
- The experience of being in hospital and undergoing surgery.
- The possibility of mutilation or, at least, of alteration in normal bodily functions.
- The social and economic consequences of the illness.

The Fact of Having Cancer

The impact of the cancer diagnosis has been discussed in the previous chapter, but needs to be mentioned in the surgical context because despair and defeatism can affect convalescence from the operation. Patients undergoing cancer surgery may manifest fear of death, fear of separation, fear of abandonment, fear of loneliness, fear of disability, fear of helplessness and fear of pain (4) and some of these fears may be especially severe in a patient with heavy responsibilities. Some patients show an initial stage of denial ("it cannot be true", "could they have mixed up the biopsy specimens" "perhaps it will go away") and this is a normal part of grief. It is .abnormal only if it continues for a prolonged period and therefore interferes with co-operation in treatment (5).

The Experience of Treatment

It is reported that those patients experiencing extreme anxiety before an operation tend to have more complications in their postoperative course (6). Surprisingly, a lack of anxiety preoperatively was also found to herald postoperative problems, suggesting that some degree of anxiety may be useful to stimulate patients to cope with the stressful situation. However, another report failed to confirm that moderate anxiety was conducive to better post-operative recovery (7).

One would expect that delay in going to the operating theatre or an unnecessarily long period of preoperative fasting would increase anxiety, but no difference was shown between two groups of 30 hip replacement patients when one group had a short period of fasting and a definite time scheduled for operation, and the other group had a prolonged fast and were told their operation would be "some time" in the afternoon (8). Both groups were, however, entered in the same intensive rehabilitation programme and this may have offset any effect from the differences in peri-operative treatment.

The Fear of Mutilation

This aspect of cancer surgery has been studied especially for mastectomy and anorectal excision with colostomy formation, as these are the most obvious and common of mutilating operations. However, less obvious operations may also be perceived by the patient as mutilation, and in some cases, hysterectomy may produce major psychological morbidity (9). Again, a patient told for instance, that "part of your stomach will be removed", may believe that he will no longer be able to eat.

High levels of psychological distress are observed following mastectomy. At one year after initial diagnosis, 25% of one series of mastectomy patients had significant levels of anxiety and depression compared with a control group who had undergone biopsy for benign breast conditions, and 33% of mastectomy patients reported sexual difficulties (10). These findings have been confirmed by other workers who also found difficulties in social adjustment, with patients being unable to return to work and withdrawing from contact with other people (11).

The assumption is usually made that this psychological distress arises as a result of the damage to the sexual self image imposed by the mastectomy and some suggest that this may be more important than the cancer itself as the major concern for mastectomy patients (12). However, a comparison of mastectomy with breast-conserving surgery and radiotherapy as the primary treatment for breast cancer showed, surprisingly, no difference in the degree of psychological distress between the two groups (13). While their mutilation is less, patients treated by breast conservation may suffer greater fears of tumour reactivation.

In our own studies, emphasis was laid on discussion of the options with the patient and participation by the patient in the decision on treatment, and little psychological disturbance was noted in either the mastectomy or the breast-conservation patients (14). Since a feeling of helplessness may be prominent in cancer patients, active participation in the decision-making process may help to reduce psychological stress.

Like mastectomy, colostomy involves major disturbance of the patient's body image. There is a less obvious sexual component to this change in body image, but the surgery involved in treating rectal cancer leads to impotence in up to half of male patients as a result of physical damage to the sacral plexus (see chapter 8). In a study of the psychological effects of colostomy, out of 57 patients studied only 3 had not experienced change in their social lives as a result of their surgery. Almost one third were still depressed at the time of study and over one half had not allowed any member of the family to see the stoma (15).

These problems appear to stem from the colostomy rather than from the diagnosis. One study compared 83 patients who had undergone rectal excision with permanent colostomy for carcinoma, with 28 patients who had undergone restorative surgery after a temporary colostomy for carcinoma. One quarter of the permanent colostomy patient were depressed and less than half ate a normal diet, but these problems were much less frequent in the other group, although the diagnosis and prognosis was similar in both groups (16). In another group of 76 patients with a permanent colostomy, 39% experienced restriction in some aspect of social life, leisure or employment. Depression was experienced by 46% and sexual difficulty by 53% (17).

Some of these problems were perceived by the patient as being due to inadequate information. More than three quarters of patients in the study felt that they were given inadequate information in hospital. One third were dissatisfied with aftercare and 17% were unskilled at appliance application on discharge. The fears expressed ranged from the expectation that the stoma would be painful (because it is red, moist and apparently swollen) to a fear of leakage in public and of an associated offensive smell.

There is a popular folklore, largely unrecognised by the medical and nursing professions, about many forms of surgical treatment and this may colour the patient's perceptions of a proposed operation. This is particularly the case with hysterectomy where fears of masculinisation may occur. Other patients are concerned that they no longer have the regular "cleanout" associated with their periods, and are worried about where the blood collects now that it no longer flows out of the body (18).

The negative feeling produced by these beliefs may be strengthened if partners also hold similar beliefs, and the myths may then become self fulfilling prophecies. Although no outward change is visible, the patient may suffer a radical alteration in their self image. To some women, hysterectomy is a "surgical disruption to the self concept of femininity" (19) and similar changes may be noted in male patients following removal of the testes. Other organs carry a lower emotional charge but may still be associated with myths which result in anxieties of which the surgeon is unaware, and therefore does not address in his explanation to the patient.

Fear of Social and Economic Disruption

A prolonged period of illness may adversely affect the patient's income, and this is often a major, but unexpressed fear for those patients who are the major breadwinners for the family (20). Patients are often surprised at the surgeon's reassurance that following surgery and convalescence they can return to normal activities because society has an image of the cancer sufferer as a permanent invalid. Associated with this economic fear is the fear of becoming a burden to the family and such a fear may become self fulfilling. Role adjustment has been noted to occur in families when the head of the family undergoes surgery for cancer. Family dynamics alter, and when previously dependent members of the family find themselves supporting the family members on whom previously they depended, this can result in marked family stress (21).

When surgery for cancer is associated with complications leading to a prolonged stay in hospital, further problems may arise. The necessarily reduced contact with the ill family member over many weeks may result in the other family members "mourning" his loss as if bereaved. In cases of prolonged hospital admission, the family may complete their period of mourning and adjust to a new life without the ill member. His return to the family circle then necessitates major readjustments, and may even result in hostilities developing. These hostile feelings are at variance with the anticipated feeling of love and joy at the patient's recovery and may lead to a sense of profound guilt in family members (22).

Patients who have undergone mutilating surgery may find it impossible to leave the house or to return to work for many months after physical recovery has taken place (16). This, in turn, may generate financial difficulties which further exacerbate the stress. Even for early stage disease, the admission of the patient to hospital may be a most disruptive factor. "The patient leaves behind a full diary and enters a world in which he sits around waiting for things to happen. All his most personal functions are monitored and are of public interest. He is often spoken to as though he had no intelligence, and as though his disease were part of the property of the hospital rather than part of himself. He presents his tumour to the hospital and hands over all responsibility for it" (23). This encourages feelings of helplessness which may subsequently lead to depression.

Coping with the Problem

Patients develop various strategies for coping with the stress of surgery for cancer but this chapter will concentrate on the strategies usedby those caring for the patient. These may be beneficial or detrimental and the latter are very often unconscious. Our aim must be to plan our approach to each patient in a way that will allow management of the physical problem with the least psychological distress.

Communication

A large element in the emotional stress experienced by the patient prior to surgery is fear of the unknown, and experiments have shown that warnings about expected symptoms from a painful episode will reduce emotional distress from those sensations. In one experiment, the painful episode was pain in the upper limb produced by inflation af a blood pressure cuff. Subjects were given either "sensory" information describing the type of pain they would experience, or else "procedural" information describing what would happen but giving no information on expected sensation. (This latter information was patterned on the typical information given to patients about to undergo a medical procedure). It was found that those patients who had received sensory information experienced less distress from the pain than those who had received procedural information (24).

A similar study was carried out in patients undergoing gall bladder removal or hernia repair. No effect was noted on the emotional response of the patients in either group, but in the gall bladder group, the patients receiving sensory information had a shorter length of hospitalisation and convalescence than the control patients (25). Studies on recovery from surgery have consistently shown that groups receiving preoperative communication have a shorter length of postoperative hospital stay than do control groups (26).

Similar benefit would result also from detailed instruction on what to expect and how to behave following discharge from hospital. Warning about expected symptoms will reduce anxiety during the recovery period, as without such warnings patients may fear that something has gone wrong when the symptoms occur. Apart from the immediate anxiety, this may lead to loss of confidence in the medical attendants and their treatment, with consequent increasing anxiety. Tiredness, tearfulness and sleeping difficulties are common postoperative problems and the patient who is told that they are a natural reaction to surgery may find them less distressing and may be more prepared to accept treatment for them.

Patients are frequently confused as to what level of activity they can undertake and how soon they can return to normal activity. Vague generalisations such as "do as much as is confortable" or "take plenty of rest" may only exacerbate the problem and most patients would prefer detailed instructions. Similarly, if patients require to take drugs or a special diet, they should learn to do this while in hospital and not have it thrust upon them suddenly on discharge (26).

Such immediate concerns are common to all patients undergoing surgery and not just to cancer patients, but in cancer patients they may be overlooked in the concern about the patient's reaction to the diagnosis. In fact, a defence mechanism on the part of some patients may be to focus on these immediate (and often apparently trivial concerns) and to ignore the more threatening implications of the diagnosis.

An example of immediate concern is that experienced by the colostomy patient. The management of a colostomy is a major difficulty for many patients and careful instruction and repeated demonstration may be necessary before the patient is competent to leave hospital and manage the colostomy alone. It is essential that the staff should be certain that he can cope and that he is confident in his coping. Patients may superficially appear to have learnt to manage their stomas, but on leaving hospital may become so underconfident as to become housebound. An early follow-up visit by the stoma therapist is necessary to ensure that all is well. There is no doubt that the increasing use of professional stoma therapists has greatly reduced the long term psychological distress of colostomy, and has also resulted in improvements in practical management of the colostomy (27).

It is important to discuss the diagnosis when mutilating operations such as colostomy and mastectomy are contemplated. Patients already perceive these operations as stating the diagnosis, and need to be able to discuss fully the implications of the diagnosis and the surgery ("will having this terrible operation save my life?"). It used to be common practice for surgeons to carry out a breast biopsy in the operating theatre and proceed to mastectomy immediately if found malignant. Two thirds of the members of the Liverpool Mastectomy Group claim that they were unaware that they were going to have a mastectomy until they woke up after the operation. Many of these women still find difficulty in adjusting to the loss of a breast and express bitterness towards the medical profession, although of course, all had signed operation "consent" forms beforehand. It may be that the population in the Group is a selected one, in that women with bad experiences tend to gravitate towards such self help groups, but nevertheless, it emphasises the need for "informed" consent in all such cases.

Counselling

In an increasing number of hospitals, a single, readily identifiable member of staff is given the task of talking with and helping patients undergoing cancer surgery. Counsellors have been most extensively used in the setting of mastectomy. It has been suggested that preoperative instruction should include a description of the operation and information on sensory effects, along with suggestions for lessening postoperative discomfort (28) which is in keeping with the studies discussed above. It is probable that the discussion should be more wide ranging than that, although many of the problems which will eventually surface will not be expected by the patient preoperatively. Contact with the counsellor must continue into the postoperative period and is discussed more fully in chapter 12.

Choice

Involvement of the patient in the decision-making process is not widespread in Britain where the traditional model of medical practice has been that the doctor makes the necessary decisions. Patients who wish to discuss their care are sometimes seen as "difficult" and some believe that to allow the patient to participate in decision-making will engender anxiety and distress or make the doctor appear inadequate. We have carried out a study on patients with breast cancer, where patients were given a choice of treatment between breast-conserving surgery with radiotherapy, and mastectomy. Contrary to our expectations, one-third of patients chose mastectomy. In those patients choosing breast-conserving surgery the chief area of concern for the patient was their appearance and body image while in the patients choosing mastectomy the chief area of concern was the diagnosis of cancer and its implications for survival and suffering. In none of the patients did any marked psychiatric problems develop (14).

Anxiety is of course produced preoperatively in the patients offered a choice but it disappears soon after surgery. The anxiety can be reduced and the patient helped to reach a decision by an informal "decision analysis" -- the patient is encouraged to examine the subjective importance and priority she attaches to the consequences of each alternative (29). It is not clear whether it is the actual process of decision analysis which produces this benefit, or the necessary investment of time by the surgeon and psychologist/counsellor. Patients express the feeling that they are being treated as responsible persons rather than ciphers.

Such clear-cut choices cannot be offered to other cancer patients where alternative treatments do not exist, but involvement of the patients in the discussion and planning of treatment is possible. Minor changes in administration of admission may allow the patient flexibility with regard to the timing of admission. This may restore some control of the situation to the patient, which may then reduce the feeling of helplessness and the consequent risk of depression. The patient must not be made to perceive themselves as a passive victim of circumstance.

Conclusion

The major requirement for the reduction of stress due to cancer surgery is awareness on the part of the medical and nursing staff of the existence of the problem and its components. Communication with, and counselling of, the patient are effective methods of stress reduction. Patient participation in treatment decisions may eliminate the feeling of helplessness which is a major component in their distress.

References

1. Carnevali, D.L. (1966) Pre-operative anxiety. American Journal of Nursing,7,1536–8
2. Lewis, M.S., Gottesman,D., Gutstein,S. (1979) The course and duration of crisis. Journal of Consulting and Clinical Psychology, 47, 128–134.
3. Gottesman D., H. Lewis M.S. (1982) Differences in crisis reactions among cancer and surgery patients. Journal of Consulting and Clinical Psychology,50, 381–388
4. Healy, J. (1970) Ecology of Cancer Patients Washington D.C. Interdisciplinary Communications Programme, The Smithsonian Institute, p.184
5. Engel, G. (1974) Grief and grieving. American Journal of Nursing, 61, 93–98
6. Janis, I.L. (1958) cited in Stress in Hospital (1979) (Ed.J. Wilson-Barnett) Churchill Livingstone, Edinburgh, p.57
7. Johnson, J.E., Dabbs, J.M.,Leventhal, H. (1970) Psychosoocial factors in the welfare of surgical patients. Nursing Research 19 (1), 18–19
8. Minchley, B.B. (1974) Physiological and psychological responses of elective surgical patients. Nursing Research 23 (5), 392–401
9. Wolf, S.R. Emotional reactions to hysterectomy. Postgraduate Medical Journal 47, 165–169
10. Lee, E.C.G., Maguire, G.P. (1975) Emotional distress in patients attending a breast clinic. British Journal of Surgery 62, 162
11. Ray, C. (1980) Psychological aspects of early breast cancer and its treatment. In Contributions to Medical Psychology, Vol. 2. (Ed. E. Rachman) Pergamon Press, London
12. May, H.J. (1980) Psychosexual sequelae to mastectomy: implications for therapeutic and rehabilitative intervention. Journal of Rehabilitation 46, 29–31
13. Sanger, C.K., Reznikoff, M. (1981) A comparison of the psychological effects of breast saving procedures with the modified radical mastectomy. Cancer 48, 2341
14. Ashcroft, J.J., Leinster, S.J. Slade, P.D. (1985) Proceedings of the Royal Society of Medicine. (in press)
15. Sutherland, A.M., Orbach, C.E., Dyke, R.B., Band, M. (1952) The psychological impact of cancer and cancer surgery. I. Adaptation to the dry colostomy: preliminary report and summary of findings. Cancer, 5, 867–872
16. Devlin, H.B., Plant, J.A., Griffin, M. (1981) Aftermath of surgery for anorectal cancer. British Medical Journal 3, 413–418
17. Eardley, A., George, W.D., Davis, F., Schofield, P.F., Wilson, M.C., Wakefield, J., Sellwood R.A. (1976) Colostomy: the consequences of surgery. Clinical Oncology, 2, 277–283
18. Raphael, B. (1978) Psychiatric aspects of hysterectomy. In Modern Perspectives in the Psychiatric Aspects of Surgery. (Ed. J.G. Howells) Macmillan, London.
19. Notman, M.T. (1976) Elective hysterectomy: pro and con. New England Journal of Medicine, 295, 266–267
20. Smith, E.A. (1976) Psychosocial aspects of cancer patient care. McGraw Hill, New York

21. Vess, J., Moreland J., Schwebel, A. (1984) An analysis of role enactment and communication in families facing cancer. Proceedings of the American Society of Clinical Oncology 3, 74

22. Clarke, A. (1983) Observations on a personal illness – a seminar. Unpublished.

23. Thompson, M.R. (1978) Communication with patients and relatives. In Oncology for Nurses, Chapter 2 (Ed B. Tiffany) Allen and Unwin, London

24. Johnson,J.E. (1973) Effects of accurate expectations about sensations on the sensory and distress components of stress. Journal of Personality and Social Psychology, 29, 710–718

25. Johnson, J.W., Rice, W.H., Fuller, S.S. Endress, M.P. (1978) Sensory information, instruction in coping strategy and recovery from surgery. Research in Nursing and Health 1, 4–17

26. Webb, C. (1983) Teaching for recovery from surgery. In Patient Teaching (Ed.J. Wilson Barnett) Churchill Livingstone, Edinburgh, p.34

27. Wilson, E., Desruisseaux, B. (1983) Stoma care and patient teaching, ibid p.95

28. Bullough, B. (1981) Nurses as teachers and support persons for breast cancer patients. Cancer Nursing 4, 221–225

29. Leinster, S.J., Ashcroft, J.J., Slade, P.D. (1985) Some critical indications for choice of early breast cancer treatment. Journal of Psychosocial Oncology (in press)

Chapter 4

Coping with Cytotoxic Therapy

ALAN COATES

Cytotoxic therapy is regarded with grave distrust by many patients, and also by a substantial number of doctors. The side effects of such therapy are real and may be severe, but they are by no means uniform in severity. Unfortunately, people often assume the worst possible side effects when decisions about chemotherapy are made. Discussion of the effects to be expected usually need to be repeated in order to overcome the communication difficulties common in patients newly aware of their diagnosis or of disease recurrence. Group discussions with other patients may also be useful, as they are in other aspects of coping with cancer (1).

Coping with Adjuvant Cytotoxic Therapy

Adjuvant chemotherapy is given with curative intent. The hope is that the use of cytotoxic drugs immediately after local treatment will improve the "cure" rate above that obtained by the local procedure alone (2)(3). The dilemma facing patients receiving adjuvant chemotherapy is that there is no evidence that their disease has spread. They will thus be aware that the local procedure alone produces some cures, and that they might indeed be undergoing the toxic effects of treatment in a cause already won. They will also be aware that the disease may recur despite adjuvant therapy, and that in this situation also, their sufferings will have been in vain. Patients must regard their therapy as a form of insurance against recurrence, in the same way that they willingly pay premiums to insure against events which may never occur.

In facing a course of adjuvant cytotoxic therapy, its finite duration is of some comfort to the patient. In the case of breast cancer where six months treatment or even less seems as good as longer periods (4, 5), patients are able to "count down" the remaining treatments. However, this can on occasion lead to so intense a concentration on the completion of therapy that the last cycle may be refused.

While most of the problems associated with adjuvant therapy disappear when the course is complete, some may persist. In a study of 35 women interviewed before adjuvant cytotoxic treatment for breast cancer and again nearly two years after treatment ended, more that half described some persisting physical problem related to cytotoxic therapy (6).

Coping with Cytotoxic Therapy for Cure of Disease

Patients with disseminated testicular teratoma, gestational choriocarcinoma, Hodgkin's disease and certain other lymphomas are among those treated with cytotoxic therapy with curative intent, even in the presence of widespread disease dissemination.

There is evidence that patients with testicular teratoma may have psychological problems predating their diagnosis. In a group of 30 patients treated at the Memorial Sloan-Kettering Cancer Center for such tumours, there was an increased incidence of prior psychiatric disturbance during puberty and adolescence, and lower educational achievement than expected (7). Such pre-existing problems may accentuate the coping difficulties of this group. The same report described an increase in anxiety, with increased frequency of consultation for minor symptoms, as patients approached the end of scheduled treatment.

Patients are usually willing to accept greater acute, or even chronic, side effects in the pursuit of cure. When such patients have some obvious evidence of disease, they naturally display a keen interest in the results of tests designed to monitor tumour response. The knowledge that cure is possible, though not certain, greatly heightens the anxiety attendant on periodic tumour response assesments.

Once the tumour response is clinically complete, their problems resemble those associated with adjuvant therapy. Surprisingly, in a study of patients responding to cytotoxic therapy for malignant lymphoma, a higher level of distress and depression was found to be associated with more rapid response (8). It was suggested that this could be due to fears that the disease, now longer visible, might progress undetected (as it had prior to initial diagnosis). An alternative explanation might be that patients experiencing dramatic tumour response may suspect that the initial diagnosis was wrong, and that they are undergoing unpleasant, perhaps dangerous, therapy for a disease they never had.

Most but not all of the psychosocial problems associated with cytotoxic therapy are limited to the phase of active treatment. However, some persist, including marital breakups occasioned by the stress of treatment. The long term physical and psychological problems after curative treatment of non-Hodgkin's lymphoma have been reported in detail (9).

Coping with Palliative Cytotoxic Therapy

In palliative treatment, the majority of patients receiving cytotoxic therapy are not curable. In these patients, treatment is given in the hope that it will alleviate symptoms of disease, although it may ocasionally be given to patients without symptoms in order to prevent or delay the appearance of future symptoms. Cost must be weighed against benefit in any decision to use cytotoxic therapy in such cases. It is rational to base such decisions wherever possible on the actual preferences of patients, rather than on excessive enthusiasm for cytotoxic therapy of one doctor, or the inflexible antagonism of another. The later part of this chapter discusses studies which involve the use of patients' perceptions in evaluating the side effects of cytotoxic therapy (10,11).

Although many patients find cytotoxic therapy unpleasant and are relieved to be given the chance to stop, other patients are reluctant to discontinue treatment because they assume that nothing more can be done for them. Some such patients may wish to participate in experimental trials: others may be better served by a frank discussion of the limitations of cytotoxic therapy in their particular case, by consideration of alternative active treatment or a program of symptomatic and supportive therapy.

Cytotoxic therapy in childhood cancer is more often given with curative intent, and at the present time is usually continued for longer than in adults. Additional side effects on growth and intellectual development must be considered. The emotional problems are shared between parents and patient to a degree dependent upon the age of the patient. There is a risk that parents will feel guilty if treatment is given, for subjecting a child to unpleasant treatment in what may be the last weeks or months of life; they may feel equally guilty if it is not given, for withholding therapy which they may later perceive as possibly curative (see chapter 15).

Patient Perception of the Side Effects of Cytotoxic Therapy

Research into the problems patients themselves associate with chemotherapy is essential if we are to achieve the best cost-benefit balance for the patient. We have carried out studies to rank in order of importance the symptoms patients attribute to chemotherapy (10). Patients were shown two series of cards, each card bearing the name of a symptom or side effect. The first series described 45 physical symptoms, such as nausea, vomiting, menstrual changes, and loss of hair. The second series covered 28 "non-physical" symptoms, including the thought of coming for treatment, effects on the family, irritability, sexual problems, anxiety and depression.

The overall ranking obtained is listed in Table 1. While the first three problems, nausea, vomiting and loss of hair were not unexpected, the prominence of non-physical problems such as the thought of coming for treatment, anxiety and depression was of interest. Despite the fact that the physical symptom cards

TABLE 1. Patient perception of the side effects of cytotoxic therapy: rank order of severity of problems (10).

1 Vomiting
2 Nausea
3 Loss of hair
4 Thought of coming for treatment
5 Length of time treatment takes at clinic
6 Having to be needled
7 Shortness of breath
8 Tiredness
9 Sleeping difficulties
10 Effects on family
11 Effects on work
12 Difficulty parking at clinic
13 Feeling anxious or tense
14 Feeling depressed
15 Weight loss

outnumbered the non-physical, 37 of the 99 patients included 3 or more of the non-physical set in their top 5 problems. Comparison of male and female patients' rankings showed that male patients ranked fear of the needle much lower than female patients, perhaps reflecting acceptable male stereotypes, while female patients were less concerned about the length of treatment.

When patients were divided according to the type of treatment they were receiving, all groups ranked nausea and vomiting as the most severe side effects, but those receiving Cisplatin gave second ranking to the thought of coming for treatment. Because of this, we have since incorporated the amnesic agent Lorazepam into the anti-emetic regimen in patients receiving Cisplatin. The only patients giving high ranking to sexual problems as a result of therapy were 40–65 year old males (10).

Measuring Impact of Cytotoxic Therapy on Quality of Life

Maguire (12) asserts that patients display a reluctance to disclose their real difficulties to the doctors providing their care. The reason may be either because they do not want to bother the doctor about anything but the provision of the best possible treatment, or because they do not perceive the doctor as interested in, or competent to deal with, their psychosocial needs. He points out the need for a practical measure of the impact of treatment on quality of life, both to compare the relative side effects of alternative treatments, and also to explore the reasons for non-acceptability of a potentially curative treatment.

Visual analogue scales are widely used in other aspects of psychological measurement (13), and have been applied to the evaluation of quality of life in cancer patients (14, 15, 16) using linear analogue self assessment (LASA) scales to monitor subjective benefits of treatment (see chapter 9). In a group of cancer patients treated by chemotherapy, we have used stepwise linear regression to examine the relationship between the patients' performance status assessed by the doctor (a measurement known to be of prognostic significance) and the patients' LASA line scores (11).

A significant relationship was found between performance status and the LASA scores for general wellbeing and pain in the group as a whole, while the LASA score for appetite was also significantly related to performance status in the patients with melanoma or lung cancer. Not surprisingly, patients' assessment of physical activity and breathlessness were significantly related to performance status as recorded by the doctor. Objective response category was significantly related to performance status, but also to the change in LASA score for pain. We concluded that the LASA scoring was both practical and feasible.

Role of the Oncology Nurse

One of the major problems identified in our studies of the patient's perception of the side effects of cytotoxic therapy was the length of time taken by treatment at the clinic. Oncology nurse specialists attached to our unit now visit patients in their homes, as well as attending clinics at the hospital. Their ability to administer some forms of intravenous cytotoxic therapy at home, limiting clinic attendances to periodic review by the oncologist, is a major step towards solving the time problems involved in cytotoxic therapy administration.

Even if funds and staffing do not permit domiciliary visits, the role of the chemotherapy nurse in the hospital and clinic setting is of great importance. In our hospital, trained oncology nurses are attached to the medical oncology, haematology, melanoma and surgical oncology units and their role is to act as first contact for most patients on treatment. They provide reinforcement of the diagnostic and prognostic information given by the consultant, review the side effects to be expected from each drug, and assist the patient by organizing diagnostic procedures in other departments.

Conclusion

The will-to-live is strong, and patients facing cancer cope surprisingly well with the frequently severe side effects of cytotoxic therapy. Doctors and other clinicians involved in the care of such patients need to assess the impact of treatment on the quality of life as well as on the length of survival. While it is necessary on occasion to encourage patients to cope with cytotoxic therapy, the more frequent and more difficult task may be to help patients cope without such treatment.

References

1. Gustafson, J., Whitman, H.(1978) Towards a balanced social environment in the oncology service: the cancer patients group. Social Psychiatry 13, 147–152.
2. Pocock, S.J., Gore,S.M., Kerr, G.R. (1982) Long term survival analysis: the curability of breast cancer. Statistics in Medicine 1, 93–104.
3. Anonymous (1984) Review of mortality results in randomised trials in early breast cancer. Lancet 2, 1205–1205
4. Tancini, G., Bonadonna, G., Valagussa, P., Marchini, S., Veronesi, U. (1983) Adjuvant CMF in breast cancer: comparative 5-year results of 12 versus 6 cycles. Journal of Clinical Oncology 1, 2–10.
5. Ludwig Breast Cancer Study Group (1983) Toxic effects of early adjuvant chemotherapy for breast cancer. Lancet 2, 542–544.
6. Meyerowitz, B.E., Watkins, I.K., Sparks, F.C. (1983) Psychosocial implications of adjuvant chemotherapy. Cancer 52, 1541–1545.
7. Gorzynski, J.G., Holland, J.C. (1979) Psychological aspects of testicular cancer. Seminars in Oncology 6, 125–129.
8. Nerenz, D.R., Leventhal, H., Love, R.R. (1982) Factors contributig to emotional distress during cancer chemotherapy. Cancer 50, 1020–1027.
9. Armitage, J.O., Fyfe, M.A.E., Lewis, J. (1984) Long term remission durability and functional status of patients treated for diffuse histiocytic lymphoma with the CHOP regimen. Journal of Clinical Oncology 2, 898–902.
10. Coates, A.S., Abraham, S., Kaye, S.B., Sowerbutts, T., Frewin, C., Fox, R.M., Tattersall, M.H.N. (1983) On the receiving end – I. Patient perception of the side effects of cancer chemotherapy. European Journal of Cancer and Clinical Oncology 19, 203–208.
11. Coates, A.S., Fischer-Dillenbeck, C., McNeill, D.R., Kaye, S.B., Sims, K., Fox, R.M., Woods, R.L., Milton, G.W., Solomon, J., Tattersall, M.H.N. (1983) On the receiving end – II. Linear analogue self assesment (LASA) in evaluation of aspects of the quality of life of cancer patients receiving therapy. European Journal of Cancer and Clinical Oncology 19, 1633–1637.
12. Maguire, P. (1980) Monitoring the quality of life in cancer patients and their relatives. In Cancer Assessment and Monitoring. (Eds T. Symington, A.E. Williams, J.G. McVie) Churchill Livingstone, Edinburgh, pp 40–52.
13. Aitken, R.C.B. (1969) measurement of feelings using visual analogue scales. Proceedings of the Royal Society of Medicine 62, 989–996.
14. Priestman, T.J., Baum, M. (1976) Evaluation of quality of life in patients receiving treatment for advanced breast cancer. Lancet 1, 899–901.
15. Priestman, T.J., Baum, M., Jones, V., Forbes, J. (1977) Comparative trial of endocrine versus cytotoxic treatment in advanced breast cancer. British Medical Journal 1, 1248–50.
16. Selby, P.J., Chapman, J.-A.W., Etazadi-Amoli, J., Dalley, D., Boyd, N. (1984) The development of a method for assessing the quality of life of cancer patients. British Journal of Cancer 50, 13–22.

Chapter 5

Coping with Radiation Therapy

ELISABETH WHIPP

A patient informed that a course of radiotherapy is needed will often react with fear and suspicion. Radiotherapy has unhappy connotations of radioactivity, nuclear power and even death ray guns! It causes radiation sickness, is dangerous, can burn and even cause cancer. Some will have had a friend or relative in the terminal stages of malignancy who has had radiotherapy, and the event may sometimes be recalled as a harbinger of death.

Books for the layman on cancer tend to underline, and frequently exaggerate, the dangers of radiotherapy. They warn that all forms of radiation are intrinsically dangerous, that normal cells are damaged and the immune system can be depressed. For the patient, side effects may sometimes be devastating and the patient feels himself at the mercy of huge inhuman machines, while staff appear to scuttle to safety behind enormous protective concrete walls.

Role of the Radiotherapist

The patient is usually first seen by the radiotherapist either following preliminary investigations or surgery. The diagnosis of malignancy has generally already been made, although the site of the primary and extent of any secondary spread may yet need to be determined. The patient may have already been told the diagnosis (often in the preceding few hours or minutes), will have deduced what the visit of a radiotherapist portends, and will be in a state of apprehension.

It may be difficult for the radiotherapist at this stage to determine the precise plan of action. Results of investigations may be awaited and social, physical and psychological factors may be hard to determine in the postoperative, anxious patient. It is necessary to explore whether the patient knows his diagnosis and its implications, and whether he wishes to know more. In practice, this is much easier in the clinic. Not only is there more privacy (patients in neighbouring beds can be prurient) but the patient is seen on much more equal terms – eye to eye, dressed, and accompanied by a spouse or friend. In addition some time may have elapsed since the shock of the diagnosis.

This first interview is taxing for the patient, and is crucial if trust is to be established. A great deal of information is imparted, although much may subsequently be forgotten or blocked. This may include a discussion about the cancer and the chance of cure, and a description of treatment and side effects.

There are two main strategies used in radiotherapy. Radical treatment is intended to cure: palliative treatment is generally used to relieve symptoms, but sometimes to prevent an undesirable development such as ulceration. Unlike surgery, where the tumour is physically extirpated, radiation leaves the normal surrounding structures more or less intact, as for example, following treatment for cancer of the larynx.

Radiotherapy is rarely given in one dose, but is fractionated into daily treatments in order to spare normal tissues, yet at the same time eradicate the cancer. The number of treatments, which can vary from one to over 35 in some cases, will depend on radical or palliative intent and also on the nature and site of the tumour. Treatment can span a few days to many weeks.

Treatment rays are just like ordinary x-rays but at higher energies: they cannot be seen or felt. The machine makes a mechanical noise when turned on, but is otherwise silent. The time the patient is left on his own is actually less for treatment than for ordinary x-rays (usually of the order of a couple of minutes) but the after-effects are quite different.

Side Effects of Radiation

The radiotherapist has to balance the beneficial effects of a course of radiation against the unwanted and deleterious side-effects. While such therapeutic equations are a basic concept in medicine, the principles of radiotherapy are unfortunately unfamiliar to most doctors. To the patient, the side effects are of the utmost concern. Specific side effects depend on the anatomical structure irradiated but it is the general subjective side effects that provoke the most anxiety, and they can be difficult to predict, even for the experienced. There is an enormous variation in side effects from individual to individual: exactly comparable treatments can prostrate one patient, while another is completely untroubled.

Radiation Sickness

Radiation sickness is a term used to describe the commonly encountered symptoms of malaise, nausea, weakness and depression. There are many different factors contributing to it, depending on which part of the body is being treated. Some sites appear to be especially sensitive, while the extremities, for example, are fairly resistant. It depends on the overall dose of radiation, the number of treatments, and the overall time over which it is fractionated. It also depends on how much of the body is treated. It is often worse when large cancers are breaking down under the impact of radiation, and is more pronounced when the patient's general condition is poor. The psychological state of the patient appears to be of some importance.

Many patients expect to feel nauseated during treatment, and it is therefore a highly infectious symptom. It is particularly pronounced when a large part of the bowel is irradiated, when it is usually accompanied by diarrhoea. Most side effects of radiotherapy are seen only after a certain cumulative dose of radiation is reached, yet nausea may follow treatment on the first day. It is generally worst in the first few hours after treatment although it can carry on into the following day, and is generally minimal after a weekend's break

The mystifying, perhaps psychological, sickness to which some are prone, is frequently at its worst on a Monday morning upon sighting the hospital and for some or these luckless few, the nausea can last for months after treatment is finished. Whether or not there is a physical basis for this affliction, it confers real suffering which cannot be dismissed. Loss of appetite is commonly associated but can be experienced even when nausea is not a problem. Taste can be disturbed by radiation, and any soreness of the mouth or oesophagus due to a local effect of radiation will make the problem worse.

Psychological Factors

It is not known why many patients undergoing radiotherapy develop weakness and depression. There are certainly physical factors involved but psychological factors also have a part to play. While the patient coming new to radiotherapy will have just learnt (or will have good reason to suspect) that he has cancer, for the patient who has been treated previously a further course of therapy means that he has recurrent or uncontrolled disease – an ample cause for depression.

Sometimes the cancer itself may be making them ill, apart from the dread of radiation and possible side effects. Many patients are admitted to the hospital for medical or geographical reasons, leading to the anxiety of being away from home and disruption of sleep pattern. In other cases travelling and the unavoidable waiting, often with desperately ill comrades, are causes for depression. There is often very little the patient can do to help himself during radiotherapy, because the disease and side effects may dominate his thoughts; however those patients with a positive attitude, through determination to fight the disease or through social support, seem to experience less general malaise.

Radiation sickness is on the whole, a rather vague and unpredictable syndrome, which is why most clinicians avoid the term. However, the misery that can be produced is an important consideration when balancing the therapeutic equation.

Prediction of Side Effects

Side effects from radiotherapy, both general and specific, are highly variable and difficult to predict. However, there are three guide-lines to the expected severity:

Dose

The dose of radiation given cannot be simply correlated to the severity of side effects: the total dose must be related by complex formulae to the number of fractions given and the overall treatment time. Although tables are available, it is difficult for anyone but a radiotherapist to compare doses and anticipate reactions. However, the bigger the equivalent biological dose, the greater the degree of the side effects.

Volume

The volume of the body treated, from the small fields used for the larynx up to whole abdominal "baths" and even total body irradiation, has a great influence on the number of side effects.

Site in the body

Some sites of the body are much more likely than others to give significant symptoms. Treatment of the extremities rarely produces malaise while the abdomen gives rise to the most problems, largely due to the amount of boweel treated.

In addition, large tumours breaking down in response to treatment cause general malaise, most noticeable in the very ill. Infection can be another important element in malaise, and diarrhoea orother specific discomforts will all add to the distress.

Management of Side Effects

Encouragement and explanation are essential in the management of all side effects of radiation, but in patients with depression, explanation and reassurance are frequently the most important factors. In serious cases, or when the sleep pattern is abnormal, antidepressants can help. For the very anxious, the use of Lorazepam, with its amnesic as well as tranquillising effects, can sometimes be justified. Support from the general practitioner can be of great importance, but sometimes psychiatric referral is necessary (see chapter 6).

Sickness due to radiation can be succesfully treated by anti-emetics by mouth or suppository. In many cases, administration of vitamin B6 (pyridoxine) can help for reasons not understood, while steroids can ameliorate symptoms in some of the seriously ill cases.

In addition to the general malaise which may be encountered, there are specific problems related to the part of the body being treated. Most are dose-dependent and develop only at critical dose levels. Some reactions are acute, developing during the course of treatment; others are chronic and become manifest many months later. In attempting to cure a tumour, both the short term and long term sequelae must be considered, and will generally dictate the dose of radiation

Skin Reactions

The reaction of the skin to radiation is dose-dependent. Modern megavoltage beams are skin-sparing, which means that the dose at the skin is only a fraction of that received some millimeters below the surface. Sometimes, a high skin dose is unavoidable, as when treating carcinoma of the larynx, because the tumour-bearing vocal cords are so near to the surface. In some cases, a high skin dose is desirable, as when treating skin cancers and mastectomy scars.

At low doses, the skin will develop redness, which becomes severe at higher doses and is followed by dry scaling. However it may progress to painful moist blistering or even ulceration especially if there is local infection or rubbing. Usually, ulceration can be avoided if the skin is observed during treatment, and treatment is suspended if the skin reaction is too brisk.

Previous or concurrent administration of certain cytotoxic drugs can make skin reactions worse as can also infection of the skin. Patients are advised to avoid rubbing the skin, which may include a ban on washing and shaving, as well as on tight clothing. Baby powder reduces friction if the skin is intact but products containing "heavy metals" should not be used during treatment as they can increase the radiation reaction.

Many different agents are used for severe reactions but gentian violet paint is often useful in encouraging the development of a protective crust. Bland ointments can be soothing. Although steroid-containing cream frequently relieves discomfort, its prolonged use can lead to long term skin atrophy. Skin treated to a high dose will suffer permanent changes of pigmentation or depigmentation and reduced blood supply, leading to poor healing if it is damaged.

Mouth and Throat Reactions

Radiation reactions in the mouth can be very painful, and prevention of fungus infections is important. Treated salivary glands tend to show diminished secretions, as do the normal mucus cells of the mouth leading to unpleasant dryness. Alcoholic spirits and smoking, because of their irritant effects, should be avoided.

Frequent mouthwashes with simple substances such as glycerol and thymol, are indicated. Anti-fungal agents are often used prophylactically, and a mild antiseptic or even local anaesthetic agent added if required. Benzocaine mucilage is helpful if eating is painful, and food may need to be liquidised. Loss of appetite may be worsened by a loss of taste, but both taste and the dry mouth should recover to some extent.

Eye Reactions

Radiotherapy will cause conjunctival reactions, and irradiation of the lens can lead to cataract. The eye is therefore avoided or protected if at all possible. Eye drops, containing antibiotics if infection is present, will help if there is a reaction. If the lacrimal glands are irradiated, it can lead to a permanently dry eye.

Bowel Reactions

The intestine generally, and the small bowel in particular, are sensitive to radiation, and diarrhoea will develop after all but the most modest doses. The severity of the symptoms varies with the amount of bowel irradiated, and if severe, can require a break in treatment. Nausea and vomiting is also dependent on the amount of bowel treated, but is much more variable.

Codeine phosphate is often a useful remedy and adequate fluid intake is of great importance. A low residue diet is recommended with the avoidance of hot spicy foods. However, if rectal symptoms predominate, menthyl cellulose or similar agents to keep the stools soft and bulky can help. Long term damage from high doses of radiation is a problem in a small percentage of cases and when affecting the rectum, chronic mucous discharge, bleeding and pain can result.

Loss of Hair

Many patients expect to lose their hair when undergoing radiotherapy, but this will happen only if the hair-bearing skin, such as the scalp, receives move than a threshold dose. Epilation is usually temporary, but may be permanent at higher doses. When cytotoxic agents cause alopecia, the hair subsequently grows well and sometimes even more thickly than before. However, following radiotherapy for brain tumours most patients will always have patchy thin hair and may need to wear a wig permanently.

Effects on the Immune System

Radiotherapy does depress the immune system to some extent but in practice, this is rarely a problem except in patients already immune-compromised, such as those with leukaemia. A fall in the number of circulating lymphocytes can be seen, especially if large volumes have been treated. Patients versed in the immune surveillance theory of carcinogenesis become very anxious about these effects, especially as to the likelihood of inducing metastatic spread. Despite some controversial papers on the subject, radiation induction of metastases has not been proved.

Irradiation of the Gonads

The effect of a low dose of irradiation on the ovaries depends on the patient's age, but at higher doses, both ovulation and the production of hormones is stopped, bringing on an early menopause, although there is sometimes a recovery. The sperm-producing cells in the testes are even more radiosensitive, and permanent sterility can result from very low doses of irradiation. The interstitial cells, however, are resistant and continue to produce male hormone. Sperm banking is offered when there is a risk of sterility. However, if the testes were not directly irradiated but received only scattered irradiation from nearby pelvic fields, there may be a degree of recovery.

Conclusion

The radiotherapist has powerful tools at his disposal, both to cure and to alleviate the effects of cancer. Good radiotherapy practice is the art of weighing acceptable risks against the advantages of treatment. Techniques and doses are not rigid, especially when palliating disease, and can often be adapted to any particular case. It is always more rewarding for the docter and less frightening for the patient if the diagnosis, aims and side effects of treatment can be freely discussed.

Students emerge from medical school with little understanding of radiotherapy, and this ignorance is general amongst the rest of the medical profession. Because professional reassurance and explanation is so hard for the patient to find, the subject is often shrouded in mystery and terror for him, when he comes for treatment.

References

1. Halnan, K.E. (1982) Treatment of Cancer, Chapman and Hall, London
2. Hall, E.J. (1981) Radiobiology for the Radiologist, Harper and Row, Maryland, U.S.A.

Chapter 6

Depression in Cancer Patients

JENNIFER HUGHES

Depressive illness and cancer are both common and frequently co-exist in the same patient. In considering the relationship betweeen them, it is important to review our knowledge of the cause of depressive illness in cancer patients, its symptoms and the diagnostic difficulties Also the prevalence of depressive illness in cancer practice and the prevention of such illness.

Defining Depression

The term "depression" is unsatisfactory because it is used for a range of states from a mild, transient variation in mood which is universally familiar, to a serious psychiatric illness which causes intense suffering and may even lead to suicide. The classification and terminology of depressive states is extremely confusing (1) and when dealng with cancer patients, a useful way of classifying depressive states is to divide them into "depressive reactions" and "depressive illnesses."

"Depressive reaction" means a lowering of mood which is obviously a response to some psychological stress. Depressive reactions may be greatly distressing but do not usually last more than a week or so in a severe form. They can best be understood as a pronounced form of normal unhappiness, as opposed to a pathological mental state. "Depressive illness" (or clinical depression) which may or may not be triggered off by external stress, involves characteristic symptoms which are rather different in quality. They are usually more severe and prolonged than the pronounced feeling of unhappiness which constitutes a depressive reaction.

Whether depressive reaction and depressive illness are best regarded as separate conditions, or whether there is a gradation from one to the other, is a matter of debate. In practical terms it is useful to separate them, because patients with the symptoms of depressive illness usually respond well to psychiatric treatment of a kind which would not be appropriate for those who were showing no more than a natural response to stress. Having said this, there is a certain overlap between depressive reaction and depressive illness, with some patients showing mixed features.

Depressive states are frequent in the general population of Western countries, especially among women. Severe depressive illness requiring psychiatric care is present in 2–4% of the population at any one time, and the prevalence of milder depressive states is between 10 and 15%.

In research, criteria are necessary to divide the population under study into those who are depressed and those who are not depressed and also to subdivide the depressed group according to the type or severity of their symptoms. The usual methods of doing this are to apply a set of symptom critera, or to use cut-off points for scores on a questionnaire. Where disorders of mood are concerned, the distinction between normal and abnormal is not clearcut, nor is there universal agreement as to how it is best made.

Causes of Depressive Illness

Both psychological and physical factors have been identified as predisposing to depressive illness. The various factors are not mutually exclusive and depressive illness in any individual can usualy be explained by the interaction of two or more factors. For example, a family history of depression, the lack of a supportive network of friends and relatives, and the presence of physical illness are all factors which are likely to increase the likelihood of a depressive illness. The following factors are known to contribute to causing depressive illness and may have specific relevance in cancer patients.

Psychological factors

A stressful life event can be identified as the precipitating cause in the majority of patients with depressive illness, although naturally, the majority of people who experience stressful life events do not become clinically depressed. In this respect, cancer patients usually suffer multiple stresses, for example on learning the diagnosis, undergoing mutilating surgery, following radiotherapy or chemotherapy with unpleasant side effects, from losing mobility and independence, suffering pain, and anticipating death.

Individuals who do not have stable, close relationships, satisfying work, adequate money or housing, are at increased risk of depression. Depressive illness can develop in any type of personality but especially in those who are habitually pessimistic who tend to have strict inflexible standards, who are prone to mood swings (cyclothymic) or are unduly dependent on others.

Physical factors

Cancer patients may have metabolic abnormalities caused by the disease process itself (like hypercalcaemia or ectopic hormone secretion) or they may be having anticancer treatments which cause mood-altering metabolic changes. Such treatments include corticosteroids, some cytotoxic drugs, and possibly also radiotherapy. Severe depressive episodes are also associated with changes in hormone and electrolyte metabolism and when such changes result from the disease or drugs, secondary depression may result.

Although in most depressed patients no structural abnormality of the brain is present, depression is a common symptom of organic brain disease from any cause. An obvious example is the presence of cerebral secondaries, but depression is not the only psychiatric manifestation here: many such patients develop confusional states, and a few become euphoric rather than depressed.

There are reports that depressive symptoms occur with unexpected frequency shortly before physical evidence of cancer manifests. This could either be because certain tumours secrete mood-altering chemicals, or because preexisting depressive states lower physical resistance to disease. Thogh both theories are proposed, neither has been proved and they will not be discussed further here.

Symptoms of Depressive Illness

Depressive illness may produce physical (somatic) symptoms which may be misleading to the clinician, (especially in advanced cancer) for they can be confused with the symptoms of the cancer process itself. For this reason, the mental symptoms of depressive illness are more valuable in diagnosis than the physical ones in the case of cancer patients.

Mental symptoms

1. *Depressed mood.* Certain features serve to distinguish depressive illness from a depressive reaction within the normal range. Depressive illness should be suspected if depressed mood seems unusually severe or persistent; if the patient describes it as having a different and more unpleasant quality than ordinary sadness (an analogy with being in a black pit is often volunteered); if it cannot be dispelled by pleasant company or diversion; or if it shows "diurnal variation," being worst in early morning and improving as the day goes on. Many depressed patients do not complain of depressed mood spontaneously, but will usually admit to it after tactful inquiry.

2. *Tearfulness.* Some patients cry at the slightest provocation, others say they want to cry but cannot.

3. *Loss of interest, inability to enjoy pleasant activities, impaired concentration.* These are valid symptoms of depression in cancer patients, but care is required when inquiring about them, for "false positive" answers may be given by patients who

are prevented from taking part in things because of physical disability, rather than from mental disinclination.

4. *Exaggerated guilt, a sense of worthlessness or being a burden to others, low self-esteem.* These are not part of the usual reaction to the stress of cancer and their presence strongly suggests depressive illness.

5. *Pessimism and hopelessness about the future, with thoughts of suicide.* Surprising as it may seem, such attitudes are not usual among cancer patients, and again their presence strongly suggests a depressive illness.

6. *Anxiety and irritability.* These are sometimes present in association with a depressive mood.

Physical symptoms

1. *Sleep disturbance.* Waking early in the morning is characteristic of depressive illness, but difficulty in getting off to sleep is sometimes also a symptom. Sleep disturbance in cancer patients may be due to depression or anxiety, but physical symptoms like pain or breathlessness are also common causes.

2. *Loss of appetite and loss of weight.* These are usual in depressive illness and also in patients with advanced cancer, so they are not helpful symptoms in distinguishing the effects of the two.

3. *Loss of energy, constant tiredness.* General feelings of being unwell are common, but are unhelpful symptoms for the same reason as noted above.

4. *Headaches, or pains in other parts of the body.* These may come into the same category as the previous ones.

There is no firm rule as to how many of these symptoms must be present before a diagnosis of depressive illness can be made, but patients who have three or four of the "mental" symptoms are almost certainly suffering from clinical depression.

Inquiry about depressive symptoms may be made by clinical interview or by a standardised questionnaire (2). Some questionnaires are designed to be administered by an interviewer, the best-known example being the Hamilton scale. Others are self-rating questionnaires which patients fill in themselves, examples being the Beck, Zung, and Wakefield scales. The General Health Questionnaire, though not specifically for depression, is widely used in surveys to detect probable cases of psychiatric illness. All these scales contain a a number of questions on the *physical* symptoms of depression, a big drawback when dealing with cancer patients. A recently-introduced alternative which avoids this problem is the Hospital Anxiety Depression (HAD) Scale (3), which appears to be the most suitable one for use in physically ill patients.

Questionnaires tend to be reserved for research work but they can be a useful aid in everyday clinical work, for example as a quick and easy means of screening all the patients in a clinic or a ward for probable depression. They are not infallible when used in this way, as they often involve crude simplification of a complex set of symptoms, and those who score highly should be further assessed by a clinical interview. A considerable number of cancer patients who are not clinically depressed show raised scores because they have marked physical symptoms, or a realistic appraisal of a hopeless prognosis. A few seriously depressed patients (perhaps because they are reluctant to reveal their distress) do not score highly on self-rating questionnaires but may be identified by a searching interview.

Prevalence of Depressive States

"How common is depression in cancer patients?" is an unanswerable question, because it depends on the site and stage of the cancer, as well as on the definition of "depression" being used. For these reasons, the exact prevalence figures obtained in different research studies vary considerably, but the same broad principles emerge. First, many cancer patients – usually about half of whatever group is being studied – do not report any significant depressive symptoms at all. Second, severe depressive illness is present in a minority, which in most studies is around 15% but ranges between about 5% and 25%. The remaining patients, say 25–45%, complain of some depressive symptoms but should probably not be classed as clinically depressed or needing psychiatric treatment.

Support for the observation that very severe depression is comparatively rare among cancer patients comes from study of their suicide rates. A large study from Connecticut (4) showed a small increase in suicide rates for male cancer patients but not for female ones. Possibly some suicides in patients with advanced cancer go unrecognised or concealed, but clinical experience suggests that this is a rare occurrence. To quote from another American study (5), in which few cases of severe depression were detected among inpatients having chemotherapy for mainly incurable cancer; "The self-esteem of the advanced cancer patient is relatively intact ... he may loathe his situation, but does not loathe himself." On the other hand, a later study on an apparently similar population found severe depression in nearly a quarter of patients (6). The first of these studies found depression was most frequent in younger patients; the second one found a strong association between depression and physical disability.

The frequency of depression in patients at an earlier stage of their disease seems to vary depending on the primary site of cancer, the nature of the symptoms and the stage of the disease when it presents. Patients with pancreatic cancer (7) and lung cancer (8) both have high rates of depression even before the diagnosis is confirmed, in contrast to patients presenting with operable breast cancer (9) who are seldom severely depressed at this time. Presumably the difference relates to the greater tendency for lung and pancreatic tumours to cause systemic physical effects by the time the diagnosis is made. In the lung cancer study, correlates of depression were the presence of distant spread, severe physical disability, and a past history of depression.

Among patients with suspected cancer for which they are undergoing diagnostic tests, anxiety is very frequent, whether or not it is accompanied by depression. Many such patients are greatly distressed by any delays in receiving a hospital appointment or learning the results of investigations. When and if a diagnosis of cancer is confirmed, some patients feel much better "knowing what they have to face up to," but others will become depressed at this stage.

Most anticancer treatments, including surgery, cytotoxic therapy and radiotherapy have been implicated in causing depression (see previous chapters). Study of inoperable lung cancer patients (10) shows that depression is more common in those not given any anticancer treatment than in those given palliative radiotherapy or chemotherapy, despite the side-effects of active treatment.

Management of Depression

Virtually all studies report that many cases of depressive illness discovered in research studies have previously gone unremarked or untreated in clinical practice. Depression is easily missed in a medical or surgical setting, as the relevant questions are seldom asked as a routine. Many patients are reluctant to "waste busy doctors' time" by volunteering psychological complaints, and the depressive process itself may render them less likely to seek help, because they consider themselves weak or worthless. As described above, screening cancer patient populations by self-rating mood questionnaires is a quick way of detecting probable cases.

Clinicians' failure to detect depression in cancer patients may be more apparent than real; they may be both aware and sympathetic, yet consider depression to be such an inevitable response to the circumstances that it does not merit comment. This attitude, though understandable, is probably responsible for much needless patient distress, for severe depressive illness usually responds well to psychiatric treatment even when there is an obvious reason for its development. Like the physical suffering of pain, the mental suffering of depression can be relieved though the underlying cancer process may be incurable.

Depressive symptoms may be secondary to organic brain disease, as in patients with cerebral metastases, rather than a psychological response to stress. Brain involvement by disease is not always obvious in ordinary conversation, but usually causes some impairment of memory and orientation which can be picked up by simple cognitive tests. Suitable tests include knowing the time of day and date; the name of the ward or clinic and the names of familiar staff; being able to repeat a fictional address or a list of five digits after the interviewer, and recalling this information five minutes later.

When depressive symptoms have been detected, and a treatable physical cause ruled out, what treatment should be given? Both physical and psychological treatments for depressive illness are available, and the two methods should be considered as complementary, rather than separate alternatives. While the majority of depressed patients benefit from some combination of the two types of treatment, it is a general rule that the more severe the depression, the more effective physical treatment by drugs is likely to be, whereas milder depressive states may respond to a psychological approach alone.

Psychological Management

A good doctor-patient relationship from the start of treatment can probably do much to prevent depression from developing. The question of whether cancer patients should always be told their diagnosis and prognosis is relevant here, and remains an issue despite the general trend in recent years for cancer to be more openly discussed, and for patients to be better informed about their medical treatment. Sometimes it does not arise; for example there can be few breast cancer patients nowadays who do not know their diagnosis, since information on breast cancer is so widely available through the media. The situation is different for some other types of cancer, including those which arise in internal organs, cause nonspecific symptoms, or tend to affect older patients from less educated social groups.

In a study of inoperable lung cancer (10) there were a number of patients who suspected their diagnosis but had not liked to discuss the subject with their doctors. Most were unhappy with this state of affairs, and this group had more depressive symptoms than those with definite knowledge of the diagnosis. Distress was particularly frequent if a relative knew the facts about the illness and the patient did not. Some cases of depression in cancer patients seem largely related to such conspiracies of silence, ending of which may lead to improvement in the patient's mood.

There is a minority of patients for whom discovery of the diagnosis and prognosis precipitates a severe depressive state. There is another minority of patients who deny any curiosity about what is wrong and seem content to remain in ignorance, though some presumably have unacknowledged suspicions of the truth. One study (11) reported that about half of a large series of lung cancer patients did not take up the opportunity to ask about their illness.

The conclusion is that cancer patients should have ample opportunity to ask questions about their illness, preferably on several different occasions, and preferably in the presence of their partner if they live in a close relationship. However, information should not be forced on those patients who indicate they would rather not know. Care in this area of patient management will often prevent or ameliorate depression.

When depressive symptoms persist, in spite of a continuing supportive relationship with those providing medical care, specialised treatment is indicated. This may entail formal counselling for patients who have marked difficulty in coming to terms with their illness; such patients frequently have a past history of psychological difficulties, or have current problems in other spheres of life.

Such management demands time; some patients respond to a single long interview but most will need to be seen on several occasions, usually for about an hour each time. The most important skills involved are the ability to be detached but sympathetic, and readiness to listen rather than give advice. Most doctors dealing with cancer treatment do not have time to provide counselling of this kind, even if they have the skill and interest required, and counselling is often best provided by other appropriately trained personnel, usually nurses or social workers. Very few cancer patients need sophisticated psychotherapy from highly trained personnel, especially as this treatment usually takes many months and can involve considerable emotional stress in itself.

Can prophylactic counselling reduce depression in cancer patients, or generally decrease their distress? The evidence on this question is reviewed by Watson (12), who examined a number of published studies in which patients given formal counselling are compared with uncounselled patients on measures of psychological adjustment (see Chapter 13). The conclusion is not clearcut; most patients who receive counselling show an improved adjustment but a minority feel worse. Presumably, if counselling is routinely given, there is a risk of disturbing the equilibrium of those patients who would otherwise successfully deny the unpleasant consequences of their disease.

In an American study (13), a third of newly diagnosed cancer patients refused the offer of counselling. Since it has been found that at least this proportion will not develop any depressive symptoms anyway, such refusals should be respected; routine psychological intervention will be unnecessary for many, and upsetting to a few. Paradoxically, however, patients who vehemently refuse offers of psychological support are often those who would appear most in need of it.

Physical Treatment

Antidepressant drugs are appropriate when symptoms of depressive illness are prominent, and they should usually be combined with a counselling approach. Amitriptyline, one of the tricyclic group, is among the oldest agents and is still widely used. It seems to be the most effective for the majority of patients, even though it can cause a number of side-effects. Dry mouth, dizziness due to postural hypotension, and constipation are frequent ones, and the drug can cause various other anticholinergic effects which require caution in patients with physical disease, or in patients in whom there is a risk of overdose. Amitriptyline can cause some drowsiness but this is often advantageous in depressed patients who nearly always have trouble sleeping, and who may be uncomfortably agitated.

The starting dose of Amitriptyline is between 30mg and 100mg daily depending on age, size and physical fitness, and for sleepless patients it is best to give all or most of the daily dose at night. If well tolerated, it can be increased to 200mg daily or more. The antidepressant effect may not show until the drug has been given for about three weeks, and it is important to persevere for this length of time, warning the patient that side effects may be troublesome at the start of treatment. These should diminish after a week or so and then the benefits should become apparent.

An alternative drug is Mianserin, which is sometimes preferred to Amitriptyline because it has fewer side effects and is safer in overdose, but it may be a less powerful antidepressant and it is more expensive. The dose schedule, and the time lag before effective action, is the same as for Amitriptyline. For patients whose depression is moderate rather than severe, it would be appropriate for oncologist or general practitioner to prescribe a course of one of these drugs, and reserve psychiatric referral for patients who do not respond.

Patients with *severe* depression should be referred to a psychiatrist sooner, for they undergo considerable suffering and are at risk of suicide, yet may show a dramatic improvement with treatment. A few such cases are best treated with electroconvulsive therapy (ECT). Despite its bad reputation, ECT is a highly effective and fast-acting remedy for severe depression, and can be safely given to cancer patients if they are fit enough for a general anaesthetic.

Conclusion

Depressive illness affects a significant number of patients with cancer. The diagnosis is easily missed, and detected cases are often not treated in the mistaken belief that depression is an inevitable reaction to the physical disease. Management should include a search for correctable physical cause, counselling patients and relatives, and a trial of antidepressant drugs.

References

1. Kendell, R.E. (1976). The classification of depressions: a review of contemporary confusion. British Journal of Psychiatry, 129, 15–28.
2. Snaith, R.P. (1981). Rating Scales. British Journal of Psychiatry, 138, 512–514.
3. Zigmond, A.S., Snaith, R.P. (1983). The Hospital Anxiety and Depression Scale. Acta Psychiatrica Scandinavia, 67, 361–370.
4. Fox, B.H., Stanek, E.J., Boyd, S.C., Flanney, J.T. (1982). Suicide rates among cancer patients in Connecticut. Journal of Chronic Diseases, 35, 89–100.
5. Plumb, M.M., Holland, J. (1977). Comparative studies of psychological function in patients with advanced cancer – I: Self-reported depressive symptoms. Psychosomatic Medicine, 39, 264–276.
6. Bukberg, J., Penman, D., Holland, J.C. (1984). Depression in hospitalized cancer patients. Psychosomatic Medicine, 46, 199–212.
7. Fras, I., Litin, E.M., Pearson, J.S. (1967). Comparison of psychiatric symptoms in carcinoma of the pancreas with those in some other intra-abdominal neoplasms. American Journal of Psychiatry, 123, 1553–1562.

62

8. Hughes, J.E. (1985). Depressive illness and lung cancer I: Depression presentation. European Journal of Surgical Oncology, 11, 15–20.
9. Greer, S., Morris, T. (1974). Psychological attributes of women who develop breast cancer: a controlled study. Journal of Psychosomatic Research, 19, 147–153.
10. Hughes, J.E. (1985). Depressive illness and lung cancer II: Followup of inoperable patients. European Journal of Surgical Oncology, 11, 21–24.
11. Jones, J. (1981). Telling the right patient. British Medical Journal, 283, 291–293.
12. Watson, M. (1983). Psychosocial intervention with cancer patients: a review. Psychological Medicine, 13, 839–846.
13. Worden, J.W., Weisman, A.D. (1980). Do cancer patients really want counselling? General Hospital Psychiatry, 2, 100–3.

Chapter 7

Denial in Cancer Patients

JENNIFER HUGHES

The mental defence mechanism of "denial" is often invoked when cancer patients appear inappropriately unconcerned or optimistic about their illness. The term is often used in a pejorative sense, but despite its potential negative consequences, denial among cancer patients can have a valuable role in enhancing both mental and physical wellbeing.

Denial and the related mechanisms are used by psychologically healthy people in everyday life; unpleasant or threatening matters are explained away or ignored altogether. Examples may be found in relatively trivial situations, like forgetting to complete an income tax form or keep a dental appointment, as well as in more extreme circumstances (for example when a devoted wife unquestioningly accepts her unfaithful husband's unconvincing excuses for frequent absence from home). The existence of popular sayings like "burying one's head in the sand," "it can't happen to me," and "what the mind doesn't know the heart cannot grieve over," illustrate denial in everyday life.

"Denial" is described in the psychoanalytic literature as one of several mental defence mechanisms which serve to protect the ego (the conscious part of the mind) against anxiety (1). Denial, which is believed to take place unconsciously without the subject's knowledge, may be defined as the rejection of a threatening aspect of reality. Several other mental mechnisms, though theoretically different from denial, may be impossible to distinguish from it. These include "repression" and unconsciously motivated "forgetting." "Suppression" is a deliberate conscious decision not to think about the threat. Most literature on cancer patients uses "denial" as a collective term to cover all phenomena of this type.

Denial and Illness

Some people deny their own vulnerability to illness, for example they may persist in smoking, drinking heavily, or playing dangerous sports because they believe that their personal good luck or outstanding stamina will protect them from the adverse consequences which may result from such behaviour in other people. Denial may also accompany physical conditions which involve direct effects on brain function, so that stroke patients with paralysed limbs may deny there is anything wrong, as may patients with dementia or frontal lobe damage.

Denial is not an all-or-nothing phenomenon, and when faced with evidence of cancer in themselves or their relatives, many people show partial degrees of denial, which may fluctuate during the course of the illness or only apply to certain aspects of it. Some writers describe adjustment to the diagnosis of cancer as progressing through a typical sequence of stages of which denial is the initial response. Again, some patients can accept only certain components of the illness, for example they acknowledge they have cancer but seem to ignore evidence that it is incurable. Others may show a realistic acceptance of the facts in the early stages, but denial sets in if their condition deteriorates later.

Some people disapprove of denial, seeing it as cowardly and weak and many psychiatrists maintain that truly satisfactory adjustment to having cancer is only possible when there is a realistic acceptance of the facts. However, denial is a natural protective mechanism, and there is evidence that it partial denial helps the patient to cope, instead of becoming overwhelmed by distress. Extreme degrees of denial, on the other hand, may be counter-productive as they may lead to poor compliance with treatment, block communication with relatives or staff, and prevent patients from organising their practical affairs or fulfilling a long-cherished ambition while they are still well enough to do so.

Denial cannot be directly observed or measured, only inferred from observation of conduct or speech. A patient is often assumed to be using denial if he asks no questions about his diagnosis and prognosis, or talks as if there is nothing serious wrong; but such behaviour also has other possible explanations. Some patients are well aware of the truth about their illness but deliberately choose to ignore or conceal it: they may wish to avoid upsetting either themselves or those caring for them, or they may simply prefer to maintain privacy (2). Such patients are using suppression, not denial. Other patients are ignorant of the diagnosis and prognosis, because they have not been explained and the signs and symptoms of their illness are too non-specific to arouse their suspicions of cancer.

In most of the literature, the presence of denial is inferred from patients' statements and behaviour and few workers have attempted systematic measurement of denial. One technique, used for a study on breast cancer patients (3) involved asking standard questions about how far the patient was able to understand and discuss the diagnosis. On the basis of their answers, patients could be allocated to one of four groups – "complete denial," "denial of diagnostic implications," "denial of affect" and "acceptance."

Patients in the study concerned were known to have been given a full explanation of their illness but in other situations, where investigators cannot be sure this is the case, the method would be less valid. Another approach which has been used to quantify denial is use of a questionnaire which assesses the discrepancy between the patient's "real" and "ideal" self (4). Though such methods cannot provide an entirely valid or comprehensive assessment of a complex psychological concept, for research purposes they are an improvement on vague subjective impressions.

It is not unusual to encounter a situation in which the patient himself is well informed and accepting about his illness, whereas a close relative is employing denial. Family communications therefore are seriously inhibited and the patient may suffer considerable distress as a result.

Staff may use denial to reduce the stress of their work. Doctors and nurses who have devoted much effort to a patient's care, invested high hopes in a new type of treatment, or become particularly fond of a patient, may deny evidence that their efforts have failed and may therefore play down early evidence of disease progression.

Denial and Delay in Cancer Diagnosis

Failure to consult a doctor as soon as suspicious symptoms occur and delaying the diagnosis of cancer until it is advanced, is often attributed to denial, but there are other explanations. Aitken-Swan and Paterson studied the reasons for delayed presentation among 314 British cancer patients (5) and found two main groups. The first group were genuinely unaware their symptoms might signify a cancer, so they did nothing until these symptoms had reached a troublesome severity. The second group suffered from fear – fear of doctors and hospitals, fear of illness in general or cancer in particular, fear of becoming dependent and having to relinquish a valued role within the family. A smaller number of patients, mostly elderly, delayed because they had a fatalistic acceptance of the diagnosis combined with a belief that no cure was feasible. Frank denial, in which the patients exhibited a bland indifference towards blatant symptoms, was cited as the main mechanism for seven patients only, but many of the rest could be said to be showing lesser degrees of denial.

In the small study of breast cancer patients mentioned above, no relationship was found between the use of denial at interview and the duration of symptoms before seeking advice (3). This unexpected finding could reflect an inevitable difficulty with studies on delay, that is, they involve retrospective assessment of mental attitude. Patients who have delayed through the use of denial have probably abandoned this psychological strategy by the time they reach treatment.

In a personal series of 33 breast cancer patients, there were 9 who had waited for 3 months or more before reporting a breast lump to their general practitioners. The operation of denial in some of these patients is suggested by statements such as "I didn't take much notice," "I hoped it would go away," "I put off coming because I felt so well" and "I don't believe in searching for things."

Denial and Knowledge of Diagnosis

Many patients with cancer do not volunteer any discussion of their diagnosis and prognosis and, as discussed above, these will include some who genuinely do not know because they have been afraid to ask or their doctors have avoided telling them; others who do know but prefer not to talk about it; and another group who are using denial to avoid being told at all, or to avoid registering the information they receive.

Aitken-Swan and Easson (6) reported on 231 British patients, selected as having an excellent physical prognosis, who were told their diagnosis by their consultant. Interviewed within the next month, 153 patients approved of being told, 44 (mostly men) "denied" knowing they had cancer, and 17 (all women) disapproved or were upset (the remaining 17 could not be classified). The findings of this inquiry, which show that most patients with potentially curable cancers appreciate knowing their diagnosis, do not necessarily extend to patients whose physical prognosis is less favourable. In a study of 183 British lung cancer patients (7) who were all given a clear opportunity to ask their diagnosis, 90 patients did ask but 10 of them subsequently showed evidence of "denying" the information. 93did not take up the invitation but 42 of these subsequently made it clear that they did know they had a fatal disease.

Denial and Treatment Compliance

The vast majority of cancer patients comply with suggested treatments even if they have not made an open acknowledgement of their diagnosis. This would suggest that denial is often only a partial phenomenon, so although a patient does not ask whether he has cancer, and talks as if he expects to recover from his illness, at the same time he readily accepts his need for a treatment such as radiotherapy which he knows is usually reserved for cancer cases.

Denial may be a factor in some patients' choice of alternative therapy for cancer. Some such patients, although they can acknowledge what is wrong with them, are unable to accept that their condition is beyond cure by conventional medicine, and may convince themselves that an alternative approach will work despite lack of evidence for its efficacy.

Denial and Depression

There is assumed to be an inverse relationship between denial and depression, since the very function of denial is prevention of psychological distress. This inverse relationship was borne out in a study of British breast cancer patients (3), in which those using denial had significantly lower scores on a depression scale than patients who accepted the diagnosis more realistically. The deniers also had rather lower anxiety scores.

In a personal series of 50 inoperable lung cancer patients (8), though no attempt at direct measurement of denial was madec patients were asked about their knowledge of their diagnosis and prognosis. None of the 19patients who said they anticipated a full recovery from their illness were clinically depressed; at the other extreme, 6of the 20patients who knew their condition was fatal had a major depressive illness. These results could be interpreted as showing that patients able to use denial are protected from becoming depressed. They might also indicate the reverse, that depressed mood prevents denial and enforces a stark appraisal of grim reality.

Denial in the Terminal Stages

In detailed interviews with 60 terminal cancer patients, only 5 spoke with absolute certainty about dying but 35 seemed aware of the possibility (9). The other 20 seemed unaware of the possibility, and ill-informed about their illness generally, but usually content with this state of affairs. These figures suggest that about a third of patients were relying heavily on denial and that more than half were using it to a limited degree, by admitting some possibility of dying but avoiding the uncompromising conclusion that death was inevitable.

A study currently in progress in Southampton is yielding similar results. A high proportion of terminally ill patients, mostly elderly and very sick, are apparently not aware how serious their condition is, and content not to ask questions. Many terminal patients have a reduced mental acuity, or are frankly confused, as a consequence of medication, metabolic disturbances or cerebral metastases. Such cognitive impairment, by clouding the perception of reality, may facilitate the use of denial.

Denial as a Successful Coping Strategy

The tendency to regard denial as a bad thing is counteracted in some recent psychological reports. Taylor (10), using interview data from breast cancer patients in the U.S.A., proposed a "theory of cognitive adaptation" to explain how surpisingly well most people can adjust to personal tragedy, or even feel enriched as a result of it. According to this theory, successful adaptation depends on denial and illusion; the capacity to distort stark facts in a favourable light. The process has three phases:

1. "Search for meaning:" most patients attributed their cancer to a specific cause,

such as mental stress or unhealthy diet, though they had no real evidence for doing so.

2. "Mastery:" two-thirds of the patients believed they could prevent a recurrence of their cancer by such steps as changing their mental attitudes or way of life.

3. "Regaining self-esteem:" after treatment many patients claimed to feel better than ever before, and tended to seek out less well-adjusted or less fortunate patients with whom they could compare themselves favourably.

The patients tended to ignore medical evidence which did not fit their theories. However, if these theories were disproved – if for example the tumour recurred despite adherence to a certain diet – patients seemed readily able to abandon their theory and find another. It seems that American cancer patients, whose culture makes it difficult for them to deny their diagnosis and its prognostic implications, still employ denial in more subtle ways to cushion the emotional impact of this knowledge.

Denial may be more frequent among older people, and in a large series of breast cancer patients where 32% of cases had delayed more than 3 months, delay was more common among older women (11). A survey in Edinburgh (12) found that many older women expressed prejudices, misconceptions and inhibitions about the practice of breast self-examination. The tendency to use denial, or other psychological barriers to dealing with cancer symptoms promptly and openly, could be natural accompaniments of ageing. Alternatively, younger people nowadays may be less prone to denial because of better education and less repressive social attitudes.

Conclusion

Should cancer patients who exhibit denial be encouraged to accept a more realistic acknowledgement of their plight? Partial denial is so common, and so often useful in enabling cancer patients to adjust to their painful circumstances, that it seems misguided to interfere. However, this needs to be qualified by a warning that apparent denial may mask ignorance and fear in patients who would welcome an opportunity to talk.

Recent court cases have highlighted the doctor's obligation to inform patients about diagnosis, prognosis, and potential side effects of proposed treatments. However, there is no current ruling to suggest that such information should be forced upon unreceptive patients. In general, a gentle counselling approach, aimed at building up the patient's trust sufficiently to permit expression of the fears which underlie the denial, is better than confrontation and challenge.

Another implication of denial comes from a British study of early breast cancer patients (13) in which use of denial was found to be associated with improved rates of survival. In this study, a "fighting spirit" was also associated with higher rates of survival whereas two other responses, "stoic acceptance" and "hopelessness and helplessness," predicted a lower rate of survival. These intriguing observations need to be replicated on other patient populations.

References

1. Freud, A. (1937). The Ego and the Mechanisms of Defence. Hogarth Press and Institute of Psychoanalysis: London.
2. Dansak, D.A., Cordes, R.S. (1978). Cancer: denial or suppression? International Journal of Psychiatry in Medicine, 9, 257–262.
3. Watson, M., Greer, S., Blake, S., Shrapnell, K. (1984). Reaction to a diagnosis of breast cancer: relationship between denial, delay, and rates of psychological morbidity. Cancer, 53, 2008–2012.
4. Levine, J., Zigler, E. (1975). Denial and self-image in stroke, lung cancer, and heart disease patients. Journal of Consulting and Clinical Psychology, 43, 751–757.
5. Aitken-Swan, J., Paterson, R. (1955). The cancer patient: delay in seeking advice. British Medical Journal, i, 623–627.
6. Aitken-Swan, J., Easson, E.C. (1959). Reactions of cancer patients on being told their diagnosis. British Medical Journal, i, 779–783.
7. Jones, J.S. (1981). Telling the right patient. British Medical Journal, ii, 291–293.
8. Hughes, J.E. (1985). Depressive illness and lung cancer, II: Follow-up of inoperable patients. European Journal of Surgical Oncology, 11, 21–24.
9. Hinton, J. (1974). Talking with people about to die. British Medical Journal, iii, 25–27.
10. Taylor, S.E. (1983). Adjustment to threatening events. American Psychologist, November, 1161–1173.
11. Nichols, S., Waters, W.E., Fraser, J.D., Wheeler, M.J., Ingham, S.K. (1981). Delay in the presentation of breast symptoms for consultant investigation. Community Medicine, 3, 217–225.
12. Leathar, D.S., Roberts, M.M. (1985). Older women's attitudes towards breast disease, self examination, and screening facilities: implications for communication. British Medical Journal, i, 668–670.
13. Greer, S., Morris, T., Pettingale, K.W. (1979). Psychological response to breast cancer: effect on outcome. Lancet, ii, 785–787.

Chapter 8

Sex and the Cancer Patient

LESLIE R. SCHOVER

Continuing sexuality is important for a man or woman facing cancer. It affirms their faith in survival. The clinician's attention to their sexual health conveys the message that the patient will survive for a while. The diagnosis of cancer also tends to make patients reexamine their priorities. Often their deepest wish is for more intimacy with loved ones. Sex is one aspect of such closeness. In short, expressing sexual feelings in spite of cancer reassures patients that illness has not taken away their vitality.

Attention to sexual health is a crucial aspect of cancer care which is often neglected. Cancer or its treatment commonly damage sexual function or cause infertility. Such problems can destroy the patient's quality of life. This chapter explores the effects of cancer on both the psychological and physical components of sexuality and concludes with suggestions for the sexual rehabilitation of cancer patients.

Psychological Impact of Cancer on Sexuality

Several emotional reactions to the diagnosis and treatment of cancer make patients and their sexual partners liable to sexual problems. They include the following:

Stress and Anxiety

Of all the psychological factors that lead to sexual problems in the cancer patient, the most common is stress and anxiety. Worries about dying from the cancer, fears of painful and disfiguring treatments, and the pressure of trying to maintain normal roles at work and in the family may be overwhelming. Little energy remains for intimacy or sexual pleasure.

Anxiety is often most intense at the time of diagnosis and treatment and at the time of follow-up appointments. Although sexuality may seem to be low on the patient's list of priorities, the clinician should use these occasions to provide sexual counseling. Many cancer centers draw patients from a wide geographic area, and patient and clinician rarely meet at less stressful times, so that sexual counseling should be offered whenever the opportunity presents itself.

Depression

Cancer patients may also be depressed. One of the signs of clinical depression is a loss of desire for sex. When patients complain of a lack of sexual interest the clinician should look for other depressive features such as depressed mood, sleep or appetite disturbance, verbal and motor slowing, a wish to be alone and feelings of guilt or worthlessness. If the sexual symptom is just part of a wider problem, it is the depression that requires primary treatment (see chapter 6).

Body Image

People who have cancer may feel less sexual because of real or imagined changes in their physical attractiveness. Many people still regard cancer as a stigma – the modern leprosy – and a man or woman may look in the mirror and see a "cancer patient" rather than a whole person. In addition, cancer treatment itself may entail temporary or permanent physical changes which may damage body image through any of the following mechanism:
- surgery that leaves a scar or removes a body part
- creation of an ostomy or the need for indwelling catheters
- radiation effects, including temporary side effects during treatment and permanent changes in skin texture or hair loss in the target area
- chemotherapy effects, such as temporary hair loss, pallor, or weight loss
- effects of hormonal therapy, including changes in fat distribution and body hair, weight gain, or the steroid "moon face."

Marital Conflict

The impact of cancer does not affect the patient alone; the structure of the marital or dating relationship is altered too. Couples who have a stable and loving relationship often feel even closer after facing the crisis of cancer (1). Relationships that will help good coping include open communication about feelings, ease in expressing affection, skill in negotiating compromises to everyday conflicts, a comfortable balance between autonomy and intimacy in the couple's relationship, and warm relations with the extended family.

Couples who were in conflict before the cancer diagnosis may, however, not be able to weather this storm. Dating couples often break off their relationship, particularly young people for whom infertility is an issue. Some married couples divorce when one partner cannot fulfil his or her expected marital roles. Sexuality cannot be separated from the context of the marital relationship. Sexual problems seem to be more common in couples who see the cancer as interfering with their relationship (1). Whether the marital conflict is cause or result of the sexual complaint is uncertain, but both need appropriate treatment.

Myths about Cancer and Sexuality

Many patients and spouses fear that cancer is contagious through sexual contact. Such beliefs are especially common when the tumor involves the breasts, genital area, urinary or digestive tracts. This myth has been strengthened by publicity about sexually-transmitted viruses and their role in causing AIDS and cervical or penile cancers. The clinician can halp a couple to distinguish between spread of cancer through sexual contact (virtually impossible) and transmission of a virus that may play a role in causing or promoting cancer.

It is also important to remind patients and partners that sexual activity in itself does not cause cancer and cannot promote a cancer recurrence. People who have experienced a sexual trauma, such as rape or incest, or who feel guilty about a past sexual experience, such as an extramarital affair or an encounter with a prostitute, are particularly likely to blame the cancer on their sexual life.

Physical Impact of Cancer on Sexuality

Many treatments for cancer may cause physiologic damage to the systems necessary for a healthy sexual response. These physical problems may affect the sexual response cycle at any of its phases (2): (a) sexual desire and the motivation to engage in sexual activity; (b) arousal involving subjective excitement, congestion of the genitals (erection in the male and vaginal expansion and lubrication in the female), and increase in autonomic nervous system functions such as pulse and respiration; (c) orgasm, i.e. the sensation of orgasm and rhythmic muscular contractions in the genital area in both men and women.

In men, orgasm itself has two phases. Emission, the first phase, is a smooth-muscle event when the bladder neck shuts tightly and peristalsis in the vasa deferens transports sperm from the epididymis to mingle with the semen emitted during contractions of the prostate and seminal vesicles. During the second phase of an orgasm – ejaculation – the seminal fluid is propelled through the urethra by contractions of the striated muscles surrounding the base of the penis. As far as is known, orgasm in women does not have two measurable phases.

A healthy sexual response requires that the hypothalamic-pituitary-gonadal hormonal axis be in balance; that the sensory, parasympathetic, and sympathetic nervous systems function properly; and that the pelvic vasculature be intact. Cancer is not the only disease that can damage these systems.

In assessing a cancer patient with sexual dysfunction, clues may be obtained from the medical history (2). Risk factors leading to sexual problems may include medications that affect either hormonal levels or neurotransmitters (e.g. antihypertensives, beta blockers, neuroleptics, antidepressants, opiates, cimetidine, and digoxin); a history of alchoholism or heavy smoking; the presence of cardiovascular disease, chronic obstructive pulmonary disease, endocrine abnormalities, renal insufficiency, diabetes, and Peyronie's disease. Women who are postmenopausal may have problems with vaginal atrophy or dryness (3). Since the majority of cancer patients are more than 50 years old, many have a history of other health problems that could affect sexual function. In addition, the specific cancer treatement may affect one or more of the various physiologic systems involved in sexual response.

Hormonal Impact

For both men and women, androgens are the hormones crucial to sexual desire (4). In women, loss of ovarian function appears to have little effect on interest in sex or arousability, as long as the adrenal glands are still functioning to produce androgens. A decrease in estrogen can lead to vaginal atrophy and dryness, however, causing dyspareunia. The hot flashes of the menopause, particularly the abrupt menopause created by oopohorectomy or pelvic radiation, may also cause enough discomfort to interfere with sexual desire (5).

Low testosterone levels in men are clearly asociated with reduced sexual desire (4). Erectile dysfunction also frequently accompanies a low level of testosterone, as does difficulty in reaching orgasm. Whether these symptoms result from a lack of mental sexual excitement or are in some way a direct effect of the hormonal insufficiency is unclear. An excess of the pituitary hormone prolactin produces a very similar pattern of sexual dysfunction in men (6), but it is not clear whether hyperprolactinemia causes sexual problems in women.

Persons with cancer may manifest hormonal abnormalities for any of the following reasons:
- radical pelvic surgery in women often includes bilateral oophorectomy
- pelvic irradiation or systemic chemotherapy may temporarily or permanently impair gonadal production of hormones
- hormonal therapy for cancers of the prostate, uterus or breast may affect sexual function
- a few tumors secrete ectopic hormones
- phenothiazines used as antiemetics, or opiates given for pain may cause hyperprolactinemia.

Vascular Impact

Damage to the pelvic vascular system affects only the arousal phase of the sexual response cycle. When a man becomes sexually aroused, the parasympathetic nervous system signals a huge increase in the speed of the blood flowing to the penis (7). Blood is shunted into the cavernous bodies of the penis, venous drainage decreases and the result is a firm erection. If the major or minor vessels of the pelvic arterial system are blocked or narrowed, a man may either achieve only partial erection or be unable to maintain erection. Arteriosclerosis in the arteries of the pelvis is probably the most common cause of organic erection problems in men older than 50. Some research indicates that defects in the venous drainage of the penis also create erectile dysfunction.

The effects of vascular damage to a woman's pelvis are still poorly understood. Theoretically, vaginal expansion and lubrication would be reduced but even in diabetic women (a group at high risk for vascular disease) the incidence of sexual dysfunction remains controversial (8).

In cancer patients a number of treatments may cause pelvic vascular damage:
- pelvic radiotherapy may cause scarring or accelerate arteriosclerosis (9)
- pelvic surgery may involve ligating minor branches of the arterial system, reducing genital blood flow (10)
- pelvic intra-arterial infusion of chemotherapy may have unknown impact.

Neurologic Impact

The exact role of the central nervous system in human sexual function remains unclear, although tumors or treatments that damage the brain can diminish sexual desire or result in inappropriate sexual behavior. Such situations are rare, however, and cancer patients are far more likely to have sexual problems because of damage to peripheral, especially pelvic, nerves. In men and women the pudendal nerve transmits sensory impulses from the genital area and is crucial to feelings of pleasure evoked by genital caressing and orgasm. The sensory nerves also control the striated muscles that contract during orgasm. The pudendal nerve is well-protected in the pelvis and is ordinarily not damaged by radical operative procedures such as abdominoperineal resection or radical prostatectomy, cystectomy, or hysterectomy (11). Even after total pelvic exenteration, both men (12) and women (13) can still feel genital pleasure and reach orgasm.

Neurologic damage from cancer treatment occurs most frequently in the autonomic nervous system. The parasympathetic nerves control arterial blood flow to the genital area and leave the spinal cord at the level of the second to fourth sacral vertebrae. In men, these nerves form a network around the prostate gland, where they are often damaged during pelvic operations such as radical prostatectomy (14), radical cystectomy, and abdominoperineal resection.

New techniques attempt to spare these nerves (15), but with the operation as previously performed, about 85% of men do not recover the capacity for full erection. Even when nerve-sparing is attempted, erections may not be recovered for six months. Men younger than 60 years (especially those under 50) are more likely to recover erections, as indicated both by Walsh (15) and by our own clinical experience with standard operative techniques. Many men can still achieve partial erection but not enough penile rigidiyy for penetration.

In women, the role of the parasympathetic nerves is not adequately studied and. Although vaginal blood flow can be measured (16), no comparisons have been made of preoperative versus postoperative flow. Nor do we know the incidence of reduced vaginal lubrication and increased dyspareunia after pelvic cancer surgery, much less the relationship between these problems and autonomic nerve damage.

The emission phase of male orgasm is particularly impaired by two cancer operations – retroperitoneal lymphadenectomy and abdominoperineal resection. Problems with emission are caused by damage to yet another component of the nervous system – the sympathetic ganglia. These sympathetic nerves leave the spinal cord at the level of the twelfth thoracic to the second lumbar vertebrae (7) and can be severed during abdominoperineal resection in the presacral area. Retroperitoneal lymphadenectomy also interrupts the sympathetic ganglia in their course along the aorta and its bifurcation into the left and right iliac arteries.

Either surgical procedure can impair emission to various degrees. In some men the prostate and seminal vesicles are completely paralyzed so that no emission occurs. Others emit semen, but the bladder neck remains open so that ejaculation is retrograde. In either situation, the man experiences a dry orgasm. Some men complain that their orgasms are not as intense as they were before cancer treatment (17). After retroperitoneal lymphadenectomy, some men recover antegrade ejaculation with fairly normal semen volume during the first 3 years after surgery (17). It is worth mentioning that dry orgasm after radical prostatectomy or cystectomy is not a neurologic effect, but rather results from removal of the prostate and seminal vesicles.

Impact of Loss of Genital Parts

Some surgical procedures for cancer remove parts of the genitals. For men, the most dreaded operations are partial and total penectomy. Partial penectomy is recommended only if the remaining penile shaft will be long enough to allow a man to direct his urinary stream away from his body. The length of the remaining penis increases with erection, so that most of these men can penetrate the vagina (11) and in spite of loss of the sensitive glans penis, orgasm and ejaculation still occur. After total penectomy, many men continue to reach orgasm through such erotic stimuli as dreams and fantasies or caressing of remaining erogenous zones (11).

In women, radical vulvectomy removes all of the sensitive areas of the external genitals, including the clitoris and labia minora. Although some women have dyspareunia because of urethral irritation or narrowing of the vaginal introitus by scar tissue, many are still orgasmic (13). Stimulation of the vagina, perineum, breasts, and other sensitive areas can increase sexual arousal and satisfaction.

A few women undergo vaginectomy, either alone or as part of a total pelvic exenteration (13). A vagina can be reconstructed, often using areas of skin and underlying muscle moved from the inner thighs and sewn together to form a vaginal tube (18). Although the skin lining the neovagina cannot produce lubrication anad never has the same sensitivity as normal vaginal mucosa, women do learn to enjoy intercourse and become orgasmic again. Many of these women still have an intact vulva, including a clitoris, but even women who had both vulvectomy and total pelvic exenteration have reported having orgasms (13).

Women who undergo mastectomy lose the erotic sensations produced by fondling the breast and nipple, and breast reconstruction does not restore normal breast sensitivity. However, breast conservation by local excision plus radiotherapy can usually preserve nipple sensation. After mastectomy, a woman's pleasure may depend on sexual stimulation to other areas of her body. Some women no longer enjoy having their remaining breast caressed after a unilateral mastectomy, but this is presumably a psychological effect of the surgery rather than an organic result.

Impact of Chronic Pain

Cancer patients may have chronic pain because of the tumor itself or as a side-effect of the cancer treatment. Whether pain occurs in the genitals or in other areas of the body, it can interfere with the ability to enjoy sexual stimulation. Often the exertion and movements of intercourse make pain more severe.

In general, men and women can time sexual activity to coincide with their periods of greatest pain relief. Often, however, medications produce drowsiness while they are at their most potent, making it difficult to feel sexually aroused. If movement or pressure exacerbates pain, a couple can be counseled about suitable positions for intercourse that minimize the triggering of pain. Genital pain, especially in women, often responds to appropriate use of lubricants and vaginal dilators (19).

Treating Sexual Problems in Cancer Patients

Little attention was paid in the past to sexual rehabilitation for cancer patients (11, 13). Sexual rehabilitation has become a more accepted part of cancer health care only as sexual attitudes in general have become more open, as success in treating cancer has resulted in long-term survival for many patients, and as treatment techniques such as sex therapy and penile prosthetics have become available (20).

Sexual rehabilitation is not merely the responsibility of professionals who specialize in sexual dysfunction. Even a clinician who is uncomfortable discussing sex should be able to bring up the topic and refer the patient to reading materials, or to other professionals for further information. Sexual side-effects of cancer treatments should be discussed, preferably with patient and partner together, when the choice of cancer therapy is being presented. We believe that an informed patient is less apt to develop sexual anxiety or to experience sexual problems than is an ignorant patient. The clinician should always stress the aspects of the sexual response that will remain normal after cancer treatment. Techniques for ameliorating sexual problems should also be described briefly at this time.

Clinicians who treat cancer patients, including physicians, psychologists, oncology nurses, and social workers, should be able to provide the following types of information and brief counseling:
- detail the effects on sexual response of the cancer treatments the patients are undergoing (1, 9–15, 17, 18);
- explain the diagnostic tests available to find the cause of a sexual problem (2, 7, 16, 19, 20);
- describe ways to cope with an ostomy appliance during sexual activity (12), to compensate for inadequate vaginal lubrication (5, 12, 19, 20), to minimize dyspareunia (12, 19), or to resume sex comfortably after an illness (12, 20);
- encourage couples to continue touching, cuddling, and non-coital caressing to orgasm, even when intercourse is not possible (12, 20).

In patients with more serious problems such as troublesome marital conflict, organic erectile problems, inability to reach orgasm after cancer treatment, persistent dyspareunia, or clear dissatisfaction with their sexual relationship, referral to a specialist may be necessary. The range of specialists who might need to be involved includes the following:
- a mental health professional who is expert in marital and sex therapy (2);
- an endocrinologist who can evaluate and treat a hormonal abnormality (3–7);
- a gynecologist who is familiar with methods of treating dyspareunia (13, 19);
- a urologist who can help couples decide whether a penile prosthesis is appropriate for them (20);
- a reconstructive surgeon who can repair vaginal scarring (18) or can restore the contours of a resected area such as the vulva, breast, or even part of the face.

Sometimes a patient needs more than one specialist. For example, a sex therapist may help a man learn to reach orgasm with a flaccid penis, so that he can make a better decision about whether a penile prosthesis could add to his sexual pleasure. A marital therapist may mediate in a couple's argument about whether the wife ought to have a breast reconstruction. It is clear that sexual rehabilitation must rely on an interdisciplinary treatment team.

Conclusion

Men and women treated for cancer are liable to sexual problems that result from a combination of emotional trauma and physical impairment. The spouse or sexual partner should always be included in efforts at sexual rehabilitation and all members of the treatment team should help in this process. Important contributions include giving the couple an opportunity to discuss sexuality and providing accurate information on the impact of the relevant cancer therapy on sexual function. The team can explain the types of resources available for sexual rehabilitation, encouraging patient and partner to resume sexual activity to the fullest possible extent. Just as psychological and physical factors combine to produce sexual dysfunction, so comprehensive treatment may involve both psychological and medical components.

References

1. Schover, L.R., von Eschenbach, A.C. (1985). Sexual and marital relationships after radiotherapy for seminoma. Urology, in press.
2. Kaplan, H.S. (1983). The Evaluation of Sexual Disorder. Brunner/Mazel, New York.
3. Leiblum, S., Bachmann, G., Kemmann, E., Colburn, D., Swartzman, L. (1983). Vaginal atrophy in the postmenopausal woman: The importance of sexual activity and hormones. Journal of the American Medical Association, 249, 2195–2198.
4. Bancroft, J. (1984). Hormones and human sexual behavior. Journal of Sex & Marital Therapy, 10, 3–22.
5. Cutler, W.B., Garcia, C.R., Edwards, D.A. (1983). Menopause: A Guide for Women and the Men Who Love Them. W.W. Norton & Co, New York.
6. Schwartz, M.F., Bauman, J.E., Masters, W.H. (1982). Hyperprolactinemia and sexual disorders in men. Biological Psychiatry, 17, 861–8876.
7. Wagner, G., Green, R. (1981). Impotence: Physiological, Psychological, Surgical Diagnosis and Treatment. Plenum, New York.
8. Schreiner-Engel, P. (1983). Diabetes mellitus and female sexuality. Sexuality & Disability, 6, 83–92.
9. Goldstein, I., Feldman, M.I., Deckers, P.J., Babayan, R.K., Krane, R.J. (1984). Radiation-associated impotence: A clinical study of its mechanism. Journal of the American Medical Association, 251, 903–910.
10. Bergman, B., Sivertsson, R., Suurkala, M. (1982). Penile blood pressure in erectile impotence following cystectomy. Scandinavian Journal of Urology and Nephrology, 16, 81–84.
11. Schover, L.R., von Eschenbach, A.C., Smith, D.R., Gonzalez, J. (1984). Sexual rehabilitation of urologic cancer patients: A practical approach. CA: A Cancer Journal for Clinicians. 34, 66–74.
12. Schover, L.R., Fife, M. (1986). Sexual counseling with radical pelvic or genital cancer surgery. Journal of Psychosocial Oncology, in press.
13. Anderson, B.L., Hacker, N.F. (1983). Treatment for gynecologic cancer: A review of the effects on female sexuality. Health Psychology, 2, 203–221.
14. Lue, T.F., Takamura, T., Schmidt, R.A., Tanagho, E.A. (1983). Potential preservation of potency after radical prostatectomy. Urology, 22, 165–167.
15. Walsh, P.C., Lepor, L., Eggleston, J.C. (1983). Radical prostatectomy with preservation of sexual function: Anatomical and pathological considerations. The Prostate, 4, 473–485.
16. Fisher, C., Cohen, H.D., Schiavi, R.C., Davis, D., Furman, B., Ward, K., Edwards, A., Cunningham, J. (1983). Patterns of female sexual arousal during sleep and waking: Vaginal thermoconductance studies. Archives of Sexual Behavior, 12, 97–122.
17. Schover, L.R., von Eschenbach, A.C. (1985). Sexual and marital relationships after treatment for nonseminomatous testicular cancer. Urology, 25, 251–255.

80

18. Edwards, C.L., Loeffler, M., Rutledge, F.N. (1981). Vaginal reconstruction. In Sexual Rehabilitation of the Urologic Cancer Patient (Eds. A.C. von Eschenbach & D.B. Rodriguez), G.K. Hall, Boston, pp. 250–265.
19. Fordney, D.S. (1978). Dyspareunia and vaginismus. Clinical Obstetrics & Gynecology, 21, 205–221.
20. Schover, L.R. (1984). Prime Time: Sexual Health for Men Over Fifty. Holt, Rinehart & Winston, New York.

PART TWO

SUPPORT OF THE CANCER PATIENT

Chapter 9

Quality of Survival –
Can we Measure it? Can we Influence it?

THURSTAN B. BREWIN

This discussion will concentrate on the quality of life in that large group of cancer patients whose outlook is neither very bad nor very good. This is a group whose chance of being in relatively good health a year after treatment is considerably better than 50:50, but that of being alive and well 10 years later is considerably less than 50:50. This type of prognosis is common in cancer and applies, for example, to the majority of patients with breast cancer.

The patient with this kind of prognosis may be in any one of several quite different clinical situations. He may have symptoms or not; his general condition may be poor or excellent; he may be in complete remission or he may show evidence of persistent cancer – slight, moderate, or gross. In addition, there may be little correlation between these three aspects, so that, for example, a patient with quite gross clinical or radiological evidence of cancer may often feel well and look well. Moreover, because some cancers are very slowly growing or even apparently static, such a person may remain well for a long time, with or without treatment.

Assessing Quality of Survival

Quality of life in any situation depends on how well we feel, how content we are, and how much we can do. All three are affected by attitudes and psychological factors, because feeling well is never purely a physical matter, and being content is never entirely psychological. Even the third factor – the ability of a person to do the things that he or she would like to do (go to work, tidy the house, take the dog for a walk, cook a meal or visit friends) is never completely physical. While doctors have always known this, recent scientific measurements have confirmed it. For example, exercise tolerance in 50 patients with chronic bronchitis was found to show a significant correlation both with measurement of mood and with certain attitudes and beliefs (1).

Peace of mind for the cancer patient depends not only on present circumstances, but also on the past (feelings of achievement or the lack of it; guilt; regrets). It depends especially on fears for the future such as fear of recurrence; of death; of unpleasant treatment; of becoming a burden to others; of being abandoned; or of leaving others unable to fend for themselves. Two patients with similar symptoms and disabilities and a similar prognosis often rate their quality of life quite differently because of different degrees of acceptance and stoicism; or different fears for the future. One may be depressed and fearful while another is optimistic, often using denial to boost his optimism.

The same is true of attitudes to the side effects of treatment such as those from chemotherapy or radiotherapy. Like the severity of cancer pain, these symptoms can never be judged purely objectively but will always depend partly on mental state and attitude. If the treatment being given is producing improvement that is obvious to the patient, then any side effects are likely to be seen by the patient in a less harsh light. Severity cannot be divorced from tolerance, nor tolerance from state of mind.

Some reported studies confirm this (2). In early breast cancer for example, when surgery has removed all evidence of disease and the patient is symptom-free, any side effects of chemotherapy will make her feel worse. Again, side effects of chemotherapy for recurrent disease that is showing no response to treatment will seem to the patient more severe than similar side effects occurring against a background of obvious benefit.

Some cancer patients go through periods of being bitter, angry, irritable and difficult to live with. One common reason is that they cannot shake off a feeling of envy for healthy people – the self pity of the "why me?" syndrome. Others, against all the odds, seem wonderfully content and grateful. They know that they may one day have a recurrence, but they will accept whatever comes.

Some patients even say that they now appreciate life more than they did before they were treated for cancer. Every day means more to them: their relationships with others seem to deepen and life is less trivial, less selfish. Soon after his 48 year old wife died of breast cancer (she had had widespread bone metastases for two years, with frequent relapses) a foreman in an electronics factory wrote, "... we were married for 26 years and if I were asked to identify the most rewarding years of our marriage I would choose the last two ... the many happy times we had during this period, realising the uncertainty of the future ...". Perhaps it is given to only a few to react to a tragic situation in this way but it does happen, and a high standard of care and moral support by doctors and nurses makes it more possible.

Then there is the problem of rapidly changing moods – even frank ambivalence. One day a patient may feel pessimistic, the next optimistic. Some will demonstrate contradictory feelings even in a single interview. One recent patient described herself bluntly as "terminal," then only a minute or two later quite spontaneously said, "I have made up my mind that I am not going to die."

Finally, if the quality of survival of a cancer patient is to be measured against the yardstick of his normal life, we have the added difficulty that normal lives vary a lot. *Before* getting cancer, the patient may have been lonely or unhappily married;

depressed or physically disabled; perhaps badly housed or in financial difficulties; perhaps suffering from problems of old age. How is this background of poor quality of life not due to the cancer to be taken into account in our assessment?

Assessment by Someone Other than the Patient

In 1948 the first index of "performance status" was introduced (3). Using a 10 point rating it aims to give an indication of what the patient is capable of in terms of general activity. The score ranges from a normal active life, through slight or severe limitation to helplessness. Since 1960 a similar but briefer 5 point rating has been preferred by many centres (4).

Such schemes give no clue as to why activity is restricted; and obviously many important points affecting quality of life are not touched on. The problem is how to give a broader picture and at the same time preserve a reasonable degree of simplicity. One such scheme (5), apparently well tested before publication, gives a quality of life score for cancer patients based on five criteria, each rated 2, 1, or 0 (top score 2). The criteria are "activity" (normal occupation, etc.): "daily living" (ability to care for self): "health" (feeling well or unwell, energy, etc): "support" (extent of moral or physical support from others) and "outlook" (mood and attitude). Full definitions for each score are given by the authors. This is an attractive scheme for the doctor in a busy clinic; the authors claim it can be completed and a total score (0–10) recorded in a median time of only one minute.

As to the purely psychological problems that cancer patients may have (for example when adjusting to mastectomy), one report has described how not only specialist nurses, but also general ward nurses, can be trained to interview patients. They may uncover hidden problems and anxieties, referring them for specialist help when necessary (6).

Self Assessment by Patients

Rather than have someone else assess quality of life, it might be thought more satisfactory to have the patient do it himself. Apart from the hope of greater accuracy, this eliminates the very real danger that others may impose their own preconceptions or anxieties into their assessment of the patient. Unfortunately, self assessment also presents severe problems, which have only been overcome to a limited extent, in spite of much effort to improve the situation (7). Patients may become irritated by questions that seem to them ambiguous or to have no relevance to their particular position. This is, no doubt, one of the reasons why many patients, when given a choice of answers, tend to go for the middle (or most "neutral") one.

Misleading or false answers may also be due to a desire not to appear uncooperative or ungrateful; or to a fear that treatment may be stopped if side effects are stressed; or to an unwillingness to admit to an increasing weakness and deterioration that is obvious to others; or, much less often, to exaggeration of symptoms in order to influence decisions or to court attention and sympathy.

The more questions there are, the less likely is the questionnaire to be completed properly, and pressure on patients aimed at improving compliance can have a serious effect on the reliability of the answers. If only, say, 60% of patients answer a particular question, can the answers received be regarded as representative?

In the "linear analogue" method of self assessment, the patient makes a mark along a line joining two extremes labelled, for example, "very well" at one end and "very ill" at the other. Some prefer this, while others still prefer the older method in which the patient puts a mark against whichever category most nearly describes how he or she feels (7, 8). A method that is particularly useful for charting the severity and duration of chemotherapy side effects is that of the Diary Card (8) in which the patient keeps a daily score for each of a number of selected criteria – for example, activity; mood; feeling well or ill; nausea or vomiting.

A number of questionnaires not intended specifically for cancer patients may also be useful. One is the Nottingham Health Profile, which assesses mobility, pain, sleep, energy, mood, social isolation, etc. (9). Sleep is particularly important to the quality of life of many patients and has perhaps been somewhat neglected in other studies. Another scheme, concerned only with mood, but much simpler and easier for the ordinary doctor to handle than the complicated methods sometimes used by psychiatrists, is the Hospital Anxiety and Depression Scale (10).

Decisions on Treatment

Mention of the word "decisions" will be enough to upset some critics, who will see it as evidence of paternalism. In this connection, it is therefore important to emphasise that: (a) the patient is supreme and can always decline our advice, but nevertheless we need to make decisions about what advice to give.(b) Patient autonomy and participation in decision making must always be accompanied by a measure of trust – the problem is *how much* participation, *how much* trust, and to what extent it is part of the doctor's job to vary the proportion of each out of respect for the feelings and personality of the patient. (c) Most reasonably sensitive and experienced doctors and nurses will agree that for many patients a direct question as to how much information they want is clumsy and inconsiderate.

All medical decisions are the result of a comparison of various options, including the option of doing nothing – or at least making no changes. To our best ability we weigh the *inherent* advantages and the *possible* advantages of each option against its inherent and possible disadvantages – all in relation to the situation of a particular patient.

There is never as much firm data about each option as we would like, so that speculation and value judgments of doubtful validity are inevitable. The problem is further complicated by unpredictable physical and psychological variations between different patients. The very same treatment that is successful in one case may completely fail in the next and there is even the risk that a treatment may actually do harm.

All this is relevant not only to the initial treatment decisions but also to the difficult problem of deciding whether or not to give patients adjuvant or maintenance therapy. Such treatment may adversely affect quality of life (2, 11). Even if we know for certain that statistically it adds a little to average survival, we cannot say whether this represents slight prolongation of life for many patients, or major benefit for a few and no benefit for the vast majority. In addition, we cannot tell who is already cured and therefore not in need of any further treatment.

Either the *quantity* or the *quality* of a cancer patient's life may be improved by treatment; and quantity covers either cure or remission. Cure can be defined in different ways. If a patient has no further symptoms due to the cancer and if the cancer does not shorten his life, there is a lot to be said for regarding him as having been cured. Remissions may be long or short, partial or complete. When a patient is in complete remission we do not know whether he is cured or not, and only by hindsight can we label him either as cured or in remission. Sometimes the evidence suggests that adjuvant or maintenance therapy is not affecting overall survival, but is increasing disease-free survival. In the wider sense of the word "cure" given above, this may increase the cure rate. This so-called "personal cure" (the patient dying of some other condition) has been studied particularly in breast cancer (12).

The other kind of benefit concerns not quantity of life, but quality. Just as morale can often be improved, so, if there are physical symptoms, it may be possible to relieve them. Many kinds of medical or surgical treatment can do this. Radiation treatment is especially useful, because it is so flexible and versatile; it can be directed if desired, only to those areas of disease causing symptoms.

Is a Grateful Patient the Best Guide?

In some ways the best indication of benefit is gratitude. Sometimes a well tolerated treatment does not achieve as many objective tumour responses as an aggressive one, but a higher percentage of grateful patients (11). However, it is unfortunately also true that in the past many cancer patients have been grateful for a treatment (surgery, radiotherapy, or chemotherapy) that was at the time thought to be beneficial (even life saving), although it was later shown to be either unnecessarily drastic or not to be prolonging life in the way that had been thought.

So patient gratitude is not by itself an adequate index of success, and we need to be sure that the gratitude is soundly based. Unfortunately, although ethical randomised treatment trials have taught us a great deal about what various treatments can do and what they cannot do, ignorance persists in several areas. The mere fact, for example, that a high proportion of a particular group of cancer patients are alive and well years later does not entitle us to regard the way they were treated as "very successful" or "very satisfactory." It may be or it may not.

The gratitude of a patient may be due to nothing more than a placebo effect, perhaps boosted to a greater or lesser degree by the powerful therapeutic weapon of suggestion. Perhaps the greatest paradox is that for some patients it is the very aggressiveness and drastic nature of a treatment that gives it its placebo effect. Doctors of compassion are concerned about the current situation in some types of cancer where aggressive chemotherapy seems very unlikely to extend worthwhile life, yet at the same time is more likely to harm quality of life than to help it. Its only rationale is to induce a feeling that "something is being done, the cancer is being fought."

Weighing Benefit against Risk

Individual variations in attitude to side effects of treatment can be very striking. Within a few hours of each other one middle aged woman said, "I don't mind vomiting, so long as I don't lose my hair" and another, "I don't mind losing my hair a bit, so long as I don't have to go through any more vomiting." Attitudes to being in hospital also vary. Some patients feel safer in hospital, others feel safer in their own home.

Equally unpredictable are attitudes to the prolonging of life. For some cancer patients, no matter what their age, life is sweet and every extra month a bonus – for which they are prepared, if need be, to pay a price in terms of side effects. Some elderly patients still enjoy life, but for others, the main reason for living is that they long to see the birth of a first grandchild or there is a distant relative that they have always hoped one day to visit. On the other hand, for some elderly patients, perhaps lonely and with nothing much to live for, a modest statistical survival advantage is of little or no importance. For them such benefit is cancelled out by even the slightest risk that the quality of remaining life might be impaired.

We must beware of too much probing in order to clarify the patient's attitude. Blunt direct questions sometimes help to clear the air but often, careful listening while watching the patient's face, is safer and kinder. We also have to be very understanding when patients show indecision and ambivalence. This is very common and is one of the reasons why many of them long for the paternalism which some well-meaning philosophers and lawyers are apparently so anxious to deny them.

Is the Specialist the Best Person to make Decisions?

When there is a difficult decision to make, should each patient have the benefit of an "advocate" – nurse, friend, personal doctor, philosopher, or ethical committee? Such an arrangement might protect the patient from a bad specialist, but falls far short of what is offered by a good one. Nobody else has the specialist's experience of benefits and side effects. Nobody else has his experience of weighing one against the other in situations similar to the one now under discussion.

The advantages in certain circumstances of very full and frank discussion with the patient are clear, and good doctors have always recognised this. The number of patients who want it has increased in recent years, even when grim alternatives, remote risks and frightening uncertainties have to be faced (13, 14). But patients have a right to compassion and common sense as well as to information and participation. Those who dislike the idea of doctors using their discretion, tend to ignore or gloss over the formidable disadvantages of injudicious or excessive attempts to involve the patient in difficult decisions. In particular, the serious risks of misconception if a patient is not accustomed to analysis; of confusion and of a sharp increase in fear, depression and uncertainty. Many friends and relatives are highly critical of those doctors who upset elderly or frightened patients in this way.

Support of the Patient

Explanation

Every patient benefits from empathy and interest and some are also helped by explanation (15). For them, at least part of the fear of what is going on inside their bodies may melt away if they hear simple explanations – not necessarily of the pathology of symptoms (talk of cells dividing and tumours growing can be very frightening to some patients) – but of their anatomy and physiology. Cancer symptoms can usually be explained in a calm matter-of-fact way. A man with shortness of breath may lie awake at night imagining cancer eating into his heart. If he hears that his heart and right lung are working normally, but that his left lung is partly out of action, he knows why he is short of breath.

If he wants further information he will either ask for it, or his manner and expression will show that he needs it. Often the protective denial mechanism – or an instinctive feeling that it might be better not to ask too many questions – will mean that enough has been said. On the other hand, the patient may accept the fact that it is cancer causing the anatomical and physiological changes described, but he prefers not to have it spelt out.

Perhaps the main question for the patient is this. Does he wish to continue being a "cancer victim", talking to his friends about it, reading books and articles on it, perhaps busy himself with some highly speculative way of fighting it (a special diet for example) in the hope of making recurrence less likely? Or is he happy to become an "ex-patient", a normal, hopeful person, not wanting to bore friends with stories of his treatment, philosophical about an uncertain future, perhaps putting into practice some preventive measure with real evidence to support it (like stopping smoking in order to reduce the chance of contracting a second tobacco-related cancer) but otherwise just hoping for the best?

The first kind of person will need a compassionate doctor – either to guide him as quickly as possible towards the second option or to be sympathetic and understanding about his desire for the first option. Otherwise he may turn to practitioners of alternative medicine, where skilled supervision may not be available and where new symptoms are less likely to be understood due to lack of basic knowledge and training.

The patient frightened about his future or by his symptoms may be helped by the comfort of touch. How badly this is needed is shown when a patient eagerly grips the hand offered him and for a moment seems reluctant to let go. Brief mention of something quite "irrelevant" and non-medical may help as an ingredient of a natural friendly relationship (15). Relatives are similarly helped by a friendly word about something non-medical, as was confirmed in one study (16). This study also had good news for busy doctors – patient satisfaction with an interview showed no correlation with its duration.

Reassurance and Encouragement

The morale of many patients with an uncertain prognosis benefits enormously when they are told of a similar patient who is now doing well, perhaps just back from holiday and enjoying life, having once been in the same position as the patient. Many patients are needlessly pessimistic, especially if elderly and in the early days after a diagnosis of cancer. They may decide that their lives are finished, when in fact there is a very real chance that this is far from being so. For them, indirect reassurance and encouragement is often more effective than direct. For example, a word about the expected frequency of check-ups ("every three months for the first two years, every six months for the next three years, then annually") or "Where are you planning to go for your holiday next year?" Some patients will react quite calmly to this – it is what they expected, they were already optimistic – but from the way others react, it is clear that they were being far too pessimistic and that encouragement of this kind was badly needed.

Some patients need a great deal of optimism if they are not to become unduly pessimistic while others need very little. There is all the difference in the world between expressions of sincere optimism and false optimism – it is mainly a matter of warmth and emphasis. Pessimism is usually bad for quality of life, whereas optimism is usually good for it. Everything possible should be done to help the patient or the "ex-patient" to get back to as full a normal life as possible. The attitude of friends and relations is important and in the fight for good quality of life can either be very helpful or very harmful.

Cancer Myths and Fears

In patients with cancer, a major factor affecting quality of survival is morale and peace of mind: abolish the element of fear and a year in remission is as good as a year cured. Some of the fears that affect cancer patients are fully justified, but many are needless or exaggerated. Reassurance of the patient may greatly improve his peace of mind.

1. A feeling that cancer is inherently horrible and unnatural. Since many cells in the body are constantly dividing in order to replace those that die, it would be surprising if the delicate balance of cell numbers did not sometimes go wrong, and a tumour result in some part of the body. In this sense cancer is no more "unnatural" than heart failure or degenerative disease of bones and joints.

2. Fear of cancer as a stigma, something shameful, perhaps even a punishment. Such conscious or unconscious fears are surprisingly common. An effective way for the busy doctor or nurse to alleviate them is to say, when talking to patients or relatives, some such remark as, "This could happen to anyone, it could have happened to me or to someone im my family".

3. Fear that the cancer might be infectious. This can lead to a couple no longer sharing the same bed; children being kept away from a sick grandparent; fear of using the same cup or the same towel.

4. Fear that the cancer is hereditary. This can lead to anxiety that cancer could be passed on to future generations, or appear later in the brother or sister of an affected child. With few exceptions, such anxieties are needless. Cancer is common and frequently, by chance, several cases appear in the same family. As with fear of infection, reassurance on this point may be received with obvious relief.

5. Undue pessimism about survival prospects. Even doctors and nurses sometimes forget that the average prognosis in a ward where every patient has cancer is often better than in a medical ward coping mainly with strokes, heart failure, advanced emphysema, liver or kidney failure and so on. "There is no reason whatever why you should not be one of the lucky ones," said with warmth and sincerity, is a useful and truthful way of helping those patients with an uncertain prognosis who are fearful for their future and who long for as much optimism as possible.

6. A feeling that long remissions in heart disease are something to be glad about, but long remissions in cancer are something to be depressed about. Heart patients accept that they are not cured while cancer patients dread that they may not be. Many people fail to see that 7 years of good quality life is just as worthwhile between the treatment of cancer and its recurrence, as it is between one heart attack and the next.

7. A fear that cancer, if fatal, is the worst way to die, more painful and distressing than other causes. In fact, in one group of 102 dying patients, physical distress persisted in 57% of patients with heart or kidney failure, compared with only 26% of those with cancer (17). Thus, we can sometimes give useful reassurance on this point to anxious relatives although with patients it is usually better not to ask directly about unspoken anxieties of this kind.

Conclusion

"In poverty I lack but other things, in banishment I lack other men, but in sickness I lack myself," wrote John Donne nearly 400 years ago. Whatever the outlook, quality of survival will depend to a great extent on how well a person can adjust to physical symptoms or disabilities, be reasonably philosophical about an uncertain future and above all, regain self respect. This can so easily get lost in the twilight world of sickness, pain, fear and indignity.

For many patients the best way to help quality of life is to do all we can to close the gap between them and the normal population. For others, whose method of coping is to join groups of other patients and spend much of their waking hours thinking of new ways to "control" their cancer (even if these ways are based on nothing more than speculation), a sympathetic doctor will do all he can to support them and supervise the situation.

We need to squeeze the last drop of benefit out of each method of treatment whether physical or psychological, and at the same time, keep an eye on the possibility of short term or long term dangers and disadvantages. Both these and the benefit need to be seen in the light of the patient's attitudes, ambitions and life style.

References

1. Morgan, A.D., Peck, D.F., Buchanan, D.R. McHardy, G.J.B. (1983). Effect of attitude and beliefs on exercise tolerance in chronic bronchitis. British Medical Journal, 286, 171–173.
2. Priestman, T.J. (1984). Quality of life after cytotoxic chemotherapy. Journal of the Royal Society of Medicine, 77, 492–495.
3. Karnofsky, D.A., Burchenal, J.H. (1948). In: Evaluation of Chemotherapeutic Agents. (Ed. C.M. MacLeod) Columbia Vincent Press, New York.
4. Zubrod, C.G., Schneiderman, M., Frei, E. et al (1960). Appraisal of methods for the study of chemotherapy of cancer in man. Journal of Chronic Diseases, 11, 7–33.
5. Spitzer, W.O., Dobson, A.J., Hall, J., Chesterman, E., Levi, J., Shepherd, R., Battista, R.N., Catchlove, B.R., (1981). Measuring the quality of life in cancer patients. Journal of Chronic Diseases, 34, 585–597.
6. Faulkner, A., Maguire, P. (1974). Teaching ward nurses to monitor cancer patients. Clinical Oncology, 10, 383–389.
7. Fayers, P.M., Jones, D.R. (1983). Measuring and analysing quality of life in cancer clinical trials: A review. Statistics in Medicine, 2, 429–446.
8. Baum, M., Priestman, T., Jones, E.M. (1979). A comparison of the quality of life in a controlled trial comparing endocrine with cytotoxic therapy for advanced breast cancer. In: Breast Cancer: Experimental and Clinical Aspects. (Eds. H.T. Mouridson, P. Palshof) Pergamon Press, London.

9. Hunt, S.M., McKenna, S.P., Williams, J. (1981). Reliability of a population survey tool for measuring perceived health problems: a study of patients with osteoarthrosis. Journal of Epidemiology and Community Health, 35, 297–300.

10. Zigmond, A.S., SMith, R.P. (1983). The Hospital Anxiety and Depression scale. Acta Psychiatrica Scandinavica, 67, 361–370.

11. Stoll, B.A. (1983). Quality of life as an objective in cancer treatment. In: Cancer Treatment: End Point Evaluation (Ed. B.A. Stoll). John Wiley and Sons, p. 113–138.

12. Brinkley, D., Haybittle, J.L. (1980). The concept of cure in breast cancer. In: The High Risk Patient with Breast Cancer. Published by Yorkshire Breast Cancer Group.

13. Cassileth, B.R.,. Zupkis, R.V., Sutton-Smith, K.m March, V. (1980). Information and participation preferences among cancer patients. Annals of Internal Medicine, 92, 832–836.

14. Ladd, J. (1980). Medical ethics: who knows best? Lancet, 2, 1127–29.

15. Brewin, T.B. (1977). The cancer patient: Communication and morale. British Medical Journal, 2, 1623–1627.

16. Korsch, B.M., Freemon, B., Negrette, V. (1971). Practical implications of doctor-patient interaction: analysis for paediatric practice. American Journal of Diseases of Children, 121, 110–114.

17. Hinton, J. (1963). The physical and mental distress of the dying. Quarterly Journal of Medicine, 32, 1–21.

Chapter 10

Types of Supportive Therapy

DAVID R. NERENZ AND RICHARD R. LOVE

Supportive therapy suitable for patients and families coping with the stress of cancer should be based on an understanding of their needs, and on the results of different approaches to meeting those needs. At present, there are few useful data in either of these areas. In the United States, supportive therapy for patients with cancer has often evolved from priorities that are not necessarily those of the patients.

In this chapter we try to make two main points. The first is that there is not a great deal known in a formal sense about what patients need in terms of supportive therapy. Although various supportive therapy programs exist, and many have done an excellent job in serving patients, most supportive therapy is not based on proven scientific studies (see Chapter 13). The second point is that the changing environment of health in the United States has had important effects on the nature of supportive therapy offered to patients with cancer. Medical care in the United States is becoming more competitive, business-oriented and cost-conscious, and this clearly places constraints on the supporting services that can be offered to patients.

The Needs of Patients with Cancer

The nature of patients' needs and the relative importance of those needs has changed as a result of changes in the care of patients with cancer over the past 15–20 years (see Chapter 1). Improved chances of long-term survival have changed the emphasis in patient needs from those of short-term prognosis, survival and religious concerns, to those of side effects of drugs, and potential for full physical recovery. The increasing use of aggressive chemotherapy also produces greater needs in areas such as inability to work during long periods of treatment, coping with side effects and susceptibility to infection. It is clear that the types of supportive therapy available to cancer patients must reflect the changing nature of treatment.

Various authors have listed areas where patients need supportive therapy. Weisman (1) lists seven areas of concern to patients, including health, self-appraisal, work and finances, family and significant relationships, religion, friends and associates, and existential concerns. He points out that many of the categories overlap. Sherman (2) has compiled a list of patient problems, including psychological issues (loss of control, denial, guilt, anger, recourse to quackery, alienation and isolation), as well as physical concerns (pain, sexual problems, and fear of recurrence). Similar lists have been published by others (3–5).

Few authors have attempted to rank order these problems in terms or their frequency of seriousness. In an analysis by Habeck (6), the basis for the rank ordering was the frequency with which 92 oncology inpatients and 106 outpatients indicated that their problems interfered "somewhat" or "a great deal" with their daily activities. A total of 85 areas of need were specified. Fatigue and inability to do heavy housework ranked as the two most frequent concerns for both inpatients and outpatients. Concerns about family and about hours worked were also mentioned very frequently by patients in both groups, while needs in areas such as understanding the illness, changes in taste, walking and ability to get around, and feeling dependent were mentioned much less frequently.

It is not clear whether patients at other institutions would have the same problems or whether different ranking procedures would produce the same results. However, an independent study using entirely different methods and a different sample of patients (although at the same clinic), also identified fatigue as the most distressing aspect of chemotherapy treatment (7).

Inquiries to a telephone cancer information service may also help to identify the relative frequency of patients' needs (8). A log of phone calls to the Wisconsin Cancer Information Service was kept to identify characteristics of callers who sought information, and to record the nature of their questions. During the period from 1979 to 1983, a total of 1226 calls were received from individuals enquiring about breast cancer. The largest number of phone calls (nearly one-third of the total) were questions on treatment and side effects. Questions on the biology of cancer and prognosis were the next largest category of questions, comprising approximately 20% of all questions from the callers.

The results of these studies suggest that issues related to treatment, side effects and ability to perform normal tasks rank consistently high in lists of important needs of patients. Information about the disease and prognosis may beless important needs to patients already well informed in this area. Most patients in the United States, particularly those treated at major cancer centers, are informed about the nature of their illness, the rationale for treatment, and the likelihood of both favorable and unfavorable outcomes. This information is provided in part by the physicians and in part by the nursing staff, and patients are usually given many opportunities to ask questions.

Such studies do not necessarily provide a list of needs of overall importance, but merely of needs *still unmet* at the time the study is conducted. Patients may have a very great need for help with religious or existential concerns, but if these needs are unexpressed or are met by clergy, social workers, or other sources, they may not be reported as needs by patients when they respond to surveys. Thus, expressed needs should be considered as important *unmet* needs rather than the most important overall need of patients.

Even if we assume that a problem such as fatigue is the single most important "need" of patients, what sort of program should be devised to meet that need? Do patients need some sort of medical treatment to make them feel less fatigued? Do they need help in organizing their affairs so that fatigue has a minimal impact on their normal activities? Do they need comfort and sympathy so that they *feel* better about their situation even if the fatigue cannot be made better and continues to have a major impact? Do they simply need information about fatigue so that they do not worry that the presence of fatigue signals a worsening of their illness?

The need for specificity in describing the needs of patients with cancer has been stressed by Meyerowitz (9). Hereports a study in which 86% of patients reported difficulty in communicating with family or friends, yet only 11% reported that the problem had to do with friends and family avoiding them. Again, patients reported a large number of different problems of communication, but only two of them were experienced by over half of the patients in the study. If one were designing a supportive therapy program for these patients, one might conclude that communication with friends and family was of such importance as to justify a major intervention effort, yet be unable to know where to start unless specific information on problems was available. Even with that information in hand, it would be difficult to design a single program that would meet the needs of more than a bare minority of patients.

Given the diversity in the problems that patients face, and the difficulty in ranking the importance of those problems, there are major difficulties in designing programs of supportive therapy that offer a package of services to a large number of patients. A more favored approach allows physicians and other members of the team (nurses, social workers, psychologists) to work individually with patients, identify specific needs, and develop strategies for solving those problems (10). Such an approach has been labeled a "problem-centered" approach (11) and describes most of the existing supportive therapy for patients.

Supportive therapy that is tailored to meet individual patient's needs requires skilled staff to identify those needs and work out plans of action. To some extent, support can be made available through outside support groups or visits from ex-patients who can answer questions from new patients (see chapter 11). When patients have long inpatient episodes as part of their treatment, it is possible to develop formal support programs that they can attend while an inpatient (12). Unfortunately, current trends in oncologic treatment and health care in general are making such opportunities less frequent and these difficultiesare discussed in the next section.

Supportive Care in Cancer Patients in the United States

Critical Trends and Changes in Care for Patients with Cancer

The last decade has seen a major change in the medical supervision of patients with cancer in the United States, in that medical oncology has emerged as the discipline predominantly involved with such patients. Up to about 20 years ago, the major treatment for cancer was surgery, and surgeons were the principal providers of follow-up and long term care of most patients. More recently there has been an increasing tendency for the co-ordination of all types of care to be conducted by medical oncologists and this has led to less prominent roles for surgeons and radiotherapists, and for primary care or general practitioners. (It should be noted that training of medical oncologists does not generally include psychosocial instruction while behavioral medicine is often part of training for primary care physicians.)

The emergence of medical oncology has resulted from the increasing availability of medical treatments for cancer. While there are some types of cancer for which clearly beneficial medical treatments are known, the availability of new drugs and preliminary reports of new approaches have led to a considerable amount of quasi-experimental chemotherapy. This situation, which lays great emphasis on *biological* treatments, has come at the expense of various types of supportive therapy, as we shall see below.

Other recent changes in the delivery of medical care in the United States are also having an unfavorable impact on the provision of supportive care for patients with cancer. Increasing concern with medical costs has led to efforts to limit inpatient hospital care. With increasing outpatient-based care in facilities not well equipped for lengthy consultations or family meetings, opportunities for good communication and supportive care are fewer. As the patient is not "captured" in a hospital room or bed for several days, social workers, educators and nurses have fewer opportunities to interact with patients.

A further aspect of outpatient-based care is that for physicians, monetary remuneration is based on what can be specifically documented to have been done for the patient. Procedure-oriented visits (for example, those where therapy of some kind of biological therapy is given) are reimbursable at higher rates than visits for supportive care. It is unfortunate also that federally-provided health insurance is in general not flexible in allowing for remuneration for time spent with patients, for whatever reasons. A final general change which is having an impact on levels of supportive care for patients with cancer, is the reduction in support by the federal government for medical research: reduction in resources automatically tends to focus greater attention on biological therapy.

These changes all lead to less time spent communicating with patients about their personal concerns. Physicians spend less time because of biological emphasis, while other health care professionals are either shut out of the outpatient system or are unavailable because of a lack of finance for their services.

There have been other changes which may be interpreted as responses to these trends. First, there have been increasingly successful efforts to promote unproven methods of cancer treatment, methods often characterized by large components of patient personal control and providing psychological support. Among the more positive responses has been the development of self-help groups, which meet to discuss a particular problem – life-threatening disease, mastectomy or colostomy. A further positive response has been the growth of the hospice movement and home care support service (see chapter 17).

Who Provides Supportive Care in Clinical Practice in the United States?

A diagnosis of cancer most commonly follows a surgical biopsy and thus a surgeon or primary care physician who arranges the biopsy will be the one to inform the patient of the diagnosis and to discuss further investigation and treatment. Increasingly, however, multidisciplinary care is proposed as the means to optimal care and medical oncologists have been championing this position. Early involvement has a positive aspect in that the medical oncologist can say that he will stick with the patient through the entire illness, for better or worse.

The primary cancer physician, (whether medical oncologists, radiotherapist, surgeon or primary care physician) usually provides or controls the professional psychological support of the patient. While some clinicians spend considerable time with their patients, particularly at times of increased anxiety (such as diagnosis, recurrence, serious illness), restrictions imposed by the outpatient nature of oncological practice generally limit this time. Those physicians with well organized practices in which nurses and other health care personnel have primary care-giving roles, may delegate much supportive therapy to such staff.

In general, we suspect that the preponderance of psychological supportive therapy for patients in the United States at present comes from nurses. In some systems (the Veterans Administration, for example) other health professionals may play a greater role in supportive care, but mostly, they are brought in only when crises occur.

The Nature of Supportive Care

The clinician's role in supportive care is to provide information, anticipate specific supportive care and counsel in crisis. The principal role is to provide accurate information to the patient about his diagnosis and treatment. Ideally this should include as much information as the patient and his family wish, provided in a unhurried atmosphere. Previous chapters have described the fears from which most cancer patients suffer, and misconceptions about prognosis, pain and the side-effects of various therapies which should be anticipated and corrected.

Participation of family members in discussions, and encouraging patients to bring written questions will both facilitate communication. Definitions of the physician's role and setting an active role for the patient in the management process are worthwhile. The major needs of patients center around getting their questions answered and a sincere effort by the physiciana to provide time for questions needs to be made.

Physicians need to anticipate providing specific supportive care which will allow the patient to function optimally, and patients need to be monitored (see Chapter 12). In general, oncological care in the United States has not been anticipatory in monitoring patient reactions or very helpful with emotional reactions to cancer. Currently, supportive care is in response to crises which come to the direct attention of the primary physician or to his staff, and their management is usually by those same people, although in some circumstances by referral to others.

Our Own Experience

As an example of patients' experiences report some of our own findings from several groups of patients receiving chemotherapy. Detailed results of these studies have been published elsewhere (13–15), but some aspects of the findings are worth mention here.

First, many patients in these studies found chemotherapy to be an overwhelming experience in the sense that it touched so many aspects of their lives. Even those patients who scored relatively low on our measures of emotional distress and who seemed to be adapting very well to therapy, could not generally forget it and get on with their lives. Many patients remarked that cancer and its treatment had become the single most salient aspect of their lives, and that it was difficult for them to think of themselves as a normal person who just happened to have an illness. Rather, they were forced to take on the role of "cancer patient."

Second, patients seemed to be less distressed by some of the very salient, acute side effects of treatment (nausea and vomiting, hair loss, for example) than by side effects which were more vague, diffuse, and systemic, such as fatigue, muscle weakness, and pain. Fatigue is very difficult to eliminate, and may last for many days, during which time it interferes markedly with performance of normal activities. While it is not as physically uncomfortable as nausea or vomiting, emotionally it seems to be more difficult to cope with.

Patients' needs for particular kinds of support will change as their clinical situation changes and as their treatment experiences change. Our data suggest that patients' needs do not necessarily reflect the seriousness of their prognosis and that patients who are likely to be cured may sometimes require a great deal of support. As an example, we noted that patients with lymphoma who had experienced a rapid and complete disappearance of palpable tumors were significantly *more* distressed than patients who had experienced a more gradual shrinkage of palpable tumors. Thus, one cannot assume that patients who are doing well medically have little need for supportive care of some kind. Other studies indicate that patients who have completed treatment and may be considered to be "cured", also have concerns, fear and needs which require supportive care (16).

Our data on emotional distress due to side effects suggest that patients may benefit by any sort of information that would allow them to clearly identify a side effect as drug-related rather than a symptom of recurrent disease. We are currently testing an intervention which provides patients with information on the nature of side effects, and by their keeping a record of side effects, may help patients see patterns in them. These patterns will help patients as they try to interpret physical sensations and organize their schedule around the likely occurrence of side effects.

In the same study, we are giving patients instruction on how to develop problem-solving skills which mayprevent or control drug-related side effects. The rationale for this approach was our observation that patients often had a great deal of information about things they could try in order to combat a side effect like nausea or vomiting, but lacked a coherent plan for knowing which to try first and how long to persist with that attempt if it did not seem to be working. Also, and how to give themselves credit for "incomplete success" rather than feeling sad or angry about inability to totally control the side effects. We have hypothesized that patients who are given help in developing integrated plans for coping with side effects will experience less distress.

Conclusion

Problems in health care delivery are playing the major role in shaping the nature of supportive care for patients with cancer in the United States. Issues such as the basis of physician remuneration and the physician's personal evaluation of various supportive efforts (reflected in the organization of personnel in his practice) are the overwhelming determinants of what kinds of supportive care patients receive. In addition, the dearth of reliable data about patient needs and results of different supportive therapies, contributes further to the limited provision of supportive therapy.

Considerable progress could be made if oncology teams spent significantly more time with their patients, as a result of which some detailed information about patients' needs would be forthcoming. However, it is more likely that the pressure for more supportive therapy will come from patient-initiated complaints, rather than from above.

With increasing treatment of cancer in outpatient settings, with increasing emphasis on biological cancer therapy, with increasing subspecialty management of patients' needs, and with a remuneration system which rewards specific procedures over psychological or other time-consuming supportive therapy, we believe that the outlook for adequate supportive therapy in the United States is very poor.

References

1. Weisman, A.D. Coping with Cancer. New York: McGraw-Hill, 1979.
2. Sherman, C.D. Coping with Cancer. In: Concepts in Cancer Medicine, Kahn, S.B., Love, R.R., Sherman, D.C. and Chakravorty, R. (Eds). New York, Grune and Stratton, 1983.
3. Coping with Cancer. NIH Publication Number 80–2080, 1980.
4. Holland, J. Psychological aspects of oncology. Medical Clinics of North Amrica, 1977, 61, 737–748.
5. Meyerowitz, B.E. Psychosocial correlates of breast cancer and its treatments. Psychological Bulletin, 1980, 87, 108–131.
6. Habeck, R.V., Blandford, K.K., Sacks, R. & Malec, J. WCCC cancer rehabilitation and continuing care needs assessments study report. Unpublished manuscript, Wisconsin Clinical Cancer Center, University of Wisconsin – Madison, 1981.
7. Nerenz, D.R., Leventhal, H. & Love, R.R. Factors contributing to emotional distress during cancer chemotherapy. Cancer, 1982, 50, 1020–1027.
8. Love, R.R., Wolter, R.L., & Hoopes, P.A. Breast cancer-related inquiries to a telephone information service. Cancer 1985, 56, 2733–2735.
9. Meyerowitz, B.E., Heinrich, R.L., & Schag, C.C. A competency-based approach to coping with cancer. In T.G. Burish & L.A. Bradley (Eds.) Coping with Chronic Disease. New York: Academic Press, 1983.
10. Goldfried, M.R. & D'Zurilla, T.J. A behavioral-analytic model for assessing competence. In C.D. Spielberger (ed.) Current topics in clinical and community psychology (Vol. 1). New York: Academic Press, 1969.
11. Heinrich, R.L., Schag, C.C., & Ganze, P.A. Living with cancer: The cancer inventory of problem situations.
12. Ringler, K.E., Gustafson, J.P. and Whitman, H.H. Technical advances in leading a cancer patient group. International Journal Group Psychotherapy, 1981; 31: 329–343.
13. Nerenz, D.R., Leventhal, H., Love, R.R., & Ringler, K.E. Psychological aspects of cancer chemotherapy. International Review of Applied Psychology, 1984, 33, 521–529.
14. Nerenz, D.R., Love, R.R., Leventhal, H., & Easterling, D.V. Psychosocial consequences of cancer chemotherapy for elderly patients. Health Services Research. (In press).
15. Ringer, K.E. Coping with chemotherapy. (Research in Clinical Psychology, No. 6) Ann Arbor, Michigan: UMI Research Press, 1983.
16. Nerenz, D.R., Leventhal, H., Love, R.R., & Easterling, D.V. Anxiety and drug taste as predictors of anticipatory nausea in cancer chemotherapy. Journal of Clinical Oncology. (In press).

Chapter 11

Help Given by Fellow Patients

H.W. VAN DEN BORNE, J.F.A. PRUYN AND K. DE MEIJ

In recent years, mutual support by cancer patients has spread rapidly. The most important characteristic of the mutual support groups is that support is given in a face-to-face contact between a volunteer and a new patient; the support is based on an exchange of their experiences.

Characteristics of Patients Seeking Contacts

In order to assess the role of help given by fellow patients, we carried out a study involving interviews with groups of patients with Hodgkin's disease (or non-Hodgkin lymphoma) or breast cancer. After the interview was completed all patients responded to a written questionnaire. In addition, interviews were held with volunteers from support groups for women who had had a mastectomy and volunteers from the Hodgkin's Contact Group. They were administered the same interview and written questionnaire as the patients, and an additional questionnaire about their voluntary work. The rationale and results of the study have been reported in detail (1–5).

By 'contact with fellow patients' we understand a form of personal contact which people have with one or more patients or ex-patients with the same illness, through a face-to-face contact or telephone conversation about problems or experiences. Of all the Hodgkin's disease patients, 51% had at some time had contact with fellow patients and the corresponding figure for the breast cancer patients was 55%. More than half of the contacts came about during a stay in hospital or at the time of the first treatment.

About three-quarters of the Hodgkin's and half of the breast cancer patients initially said that they would like to know more about how others react to their illness and its treatment, and it was expected that this need for social comparison would be reflected in actual contact with fellow patients. However, this appeared to be the case for only about half of the patients. Perhaps some of the patients satisfy their need for comparison with fellow patients in other ways (for example by reading about them) or it is possible that they simply do not know any fellow patients. Thus, only about a quarter of the patients were expressing a wish to come into contact with fellow patients.

We found that patients who want to compare their situation with that of fellow patients experience more uncertainty compared with those who have no need for comparison. Also they are more afraid of the progress of the disease and of its personal and social consequences. Furthermore, they stated that they had recently paid more attention to obtaining more information about their disease, to their relations with others and to helping others with their problems.

Breast cancer patients who had actually made contact with fellow patients differed from those who had not, in that they were less inclined to resign themselves, and more inclined to go and talk with experts and people in their immediate environment when confronted with problems relating to their illness. Hodgkin's patients who actually made contact with fellow patients differed from those who had not, in that they ascribed relatively more influence over the course of the illness to themselves. Although there is a difference between breast cancer patients and patients with Hodgkin's disease, it can be concluded that patients' coping strategies affect their decision whether or not to make contact with fellow sufferers.

About half of both groups who had had contact with fellow patients reported that contact was meaningful for themselves. Two thirds of the Hodgkin's patients and three quarters of the breast cancer patients were satisfied with the contacts with volunteers or contact persons, or with fellow patients who were neither volunteers nor contact persons. Other subjective evaluations of contact with fellow sufferers can be summarized as follows:
- about one third who had contact with fellow patients reported that they knew more about their illness and treatment as a result of that contact (reduction of uncertainty);
- about one third reported that they felt less anxious and about one half reported that they felt better as a result of contact with a fellow patient (reduction of negative feelings);
- about half reported that they experienced more grip on their situation as a result of the contact (reduction of loss of control);
- about half reported that contact with a fellow sufferer affirmed their self-esteem;
- three quarters of all patients reported that by contact with a fellow-sufferer they realised that they were not the only ones with feelings of anxiety and uncertainty. Recognition and acknowledgement of each others' problems appears to be essential in the contact between patients and ex-patients. It seems that contact with fellow sufferers gives the patients a better perspective of their own situation.

Other Studies on Mutual Support Groups

This review refers only to published studies on the effects of interaction between patients. Most of these studies consider group meetings as the main characteristics of mutual support, and only a few studies consider face-to-face contact between the ex-patient/volunteer and the new patient (6–12). If the emphasis has been on educational information programs or on counselling by a psychologist or group leader, the studies have not been included in this review. We found only 15 studies which met the criteria mentioned (6–20).

Most of these studies can hardly be compared to one another due to the variety of research methods. Only five studies (9, 10, 13–15) used a control group and only three of these studies randomized the patients. Only four studies mention a theoretical base for their research (10, 11, 15, 16). Half of the studies (9, 10, 12, 14–18) concern breast cancer patients while the others concern Hodgkin's disease (13), ostomy (11), leukemia (19) or a mixture of cancer patients (6–9, 20).

If we list the effects of contact with fellow-sufferers, it is striking that all studies but one mention positive benefit. Cancer patients feel less uncertain (17); they experience less depression and other negative feelings (17); they have a greater chance of accepting themselves (9, 10, 14, 18); they report feeling better able to cope with the disease (8, 9). Patients who take part in self-help groups have more activities than those who don't attend self-help groups (12, 16); there is better communication about their illness at home (16, 18–20). Some studies don't specify the benefit experienced, but conclude that patients are positive about the experience (6, 7, 15). Two studies (6, 13) don't find any benefit from a self-help group in comparison to a control group.

Patient Problems and Coping Strategies

The benefits from mutual help can be related to the main problems of cancer patients. These can be summarized under four headings:

1. **Uncertainty**, defined as the experience of a lack of information regarding an important value-system of the individual. We found that the majority of patients with Hodgkin's disease or breast cancer had a strong desire to know more about the cause of their illness. The next most frequently expressed areas of uncertainty were the possible consequences of the illness, the results of treatment and the necessity or purpose of treatment.

2. **Negative feelings** in cancer patients are commonly anxiety and feelings of depression, but other negative feelings are loneliness, shame, feelings of helplessness and hopelessness. In our study we found that about three-quarters of the patients were afraid that the illness would recur and many patients were apprehensive about undergoing new treatment, about becoming dependent on other people, and afraid of dying. Other frequently mentioned negative feelings were tiredness, worrying and irritability. About one third of all patients felt desperate about the future.

3. **Loss of control**, defined as the inability to manage or influence events. Loss

of control can be experienced in a number of daily events, for example, admission to a hospital and submission to unfamiliar rules. Physical, financial and related losses can also lead to a feeling of loss of control. The patient may feel that he no longer has a grip on his own situation and cannot make plans for the future. Results of the study indicate that more than half of the patients reported that because of their illness they no longer felt 'quite themselves,' an indication of loss of control. Furthermore, about half of the patients reported that they were no longer able to do what they used to do in their spare time or at work.

4. **Threat to self-esteem** is an important consequence of cancer and cancer treatment. A patient whose self-esteem had previously always been based on his own body, his achievements and his relations with others, may feel his self-esteem threatened when cancer has been diagnosed. In our study we found that up to one half of the patients believed that they had become less physically attractive since their illness or treatment.

When confronted with these feelings, cancer patients strive for a reduction or elimination of the problems. Individuals use different means in order to reduce uncertainty and negative feelings, to gain some control over the situation and to maintain self-esteem. The following major coping strategies can be distinguished:

1. **Seeking information** is a strategy primarily used to reduce uncertainty; other negative feelings such as fear can also be reduced by information. Social comparison theory (21) proposes that people prefer to try to reduce their feelings of uncertainty by means of objective information ('hard' facts) from experts such as the doctor who is treating them.

In our study we found that about half of the patients reported that they would talk to their medical specialist in case of problems, while a small proportion who indicated that they would talk to fellow patients, received most of the important information from him; about half of the patients received it from literature or from a library; while only a small minority obtained it from fellow patients (22).

2. **Seeking support and comfort** is a strategy often used to reduce negative feelings, and Schachter (21) found that people in a threatening situation prefer to be with others who are in a comparable situation. We found that a very high proportion of the patients tended to go and talk with their marital partner in case of problems and that the partner was their most important source of support. Only one in four patients said that they had received important support from a fellow-patient. Seeking support and comfort can also take place in religion, and about half of the patients reported that they seek comfort in their religion when they experience problems and most seek strength in prayer in such circumstances.

3. **Attribution** is an important coping strategy in cancer patients (23) in that people tend to see reality in their own way and to give it their own special meaning. They do this by attributing causes, for example, by blaming something or somebody. Through this process one reduces uncertainty and may feel more control over the situation. In our study more than 80% of the patients attributed the cause of their

illness to chance, and only one out of seven patients believed that they themselves or their life-style were responsible for the cause of their illness. With respect to the course of the illness, a very high proportion of patients believed that they could exert some influence on its course, while two thirds believed that God could influence the course of the illness.

4. **Denial and avoiding confrontation** are frequent in cancer patients (see Chapter 7). They are primarily used to prevent negative feelings and to protect self-esteem. Denial presumes a lack of awareness of relevant aspects of the illness while avoidance implies that the individual is aware of them but tries to suppress them or avoid confrontation with the implications. We found that a large majority of patients try to forget as quickly as possible when they are confronted with uncertainty, negative feelings or loss of control.

5. **Active coping strategy** involves seeking actively for possible ways to improve the situation by rational thought.

6. **Acceptance**. More than half of the patients stated that they resign themselves to negative feelings if confronted with them and that they take a 'wait'n see' attitude in such circumstances.

7. **Impulsive action**. Getting angry or crying was a means of coping with very intensive negative feelings or loss of control.

Activities and Motivation of Volunteers

The major activity of the volunteer is in giving support to new cancer patients in individual face-to-face contacts. This individual support can take place in the hospital but more usually it takes place in the patient's home or the home of the volunteer. The second most important activity is knowledge dissemination by giving lectures, composing a contact-bulletin or by patient representation. Lectures are given to medical students, student nurses, women's organisations and others about problems of cancer patients, organization of the volunteer work, breast-self examination, problems in aftercare, or about one's own experience as a cancer patient. Representation of the patient may be necessary with respect to physicians, hospitals, insurance companies and so on.

A third group of activities involves helping patients by means of organised activities. About half of the volunteers take part in an organised telephone support service at regular times. Also, about one third of the volunteers directly offer help by means of coaching or organising encounter groups, and by organising contact meetings for patients and their families and friends. Other activities performed by volunteers include administrative work, helping the patient during treatment (e.g. by accompanying her to the hospital), helping the patient with financial and material problems or mediating in such problems, and coaching at a physical exercise club (e.g. a gymnastic or swimming club).

The individual motivation for doing volunteer work is a combination of different reasons. The strongest reported by nearly every volunteer is the wish to help new patients and this motive is strongly coloured by idealism. The second most frequently mentioned motive is that the volunteer feels that professionals fall short of meeting important needs of patients. Some volunteers think that the professional cannot meet the needs of patients because they cannot share the same experiences, or that professionals don't have enough time for helping and supporting the patient adequately. Three quarters of the volunteers reported as an important reason that professionals are sometimes inadequate, while over half said that their own negative experience was an important motive.

A third motive is the perspective which the volunteers gain for their own personal development or recovery. Over one third of the volunteers consider this to be important. They say that by means of this work you get information that is important for yourself, and that through this work you are better able to solve your own problems. A fourth factor that plays a part in the motivation of volunteers is the distraction that is found in volunteering. Up to one quarter reported that 'to have something to do' is an important reason for working as a volunteer. The last two motives indicate that by giving help, the volunteer herself is also helped.

Riessman (24) introduced the term 'helper-therapy principle' meaning that the helper often profits more than the helped. Our study shows that over one third of volunteers report that their personal development or their own recovery is an important motive for volunteer work. Another finding was that over half the patients who had had contact with fellow patients who were not volunteers reported that they had been able to help the other person with certain problems.

One can ask therefore, what is the difference between helpers (volunteers) and helped ones. The most important differences between volunteers and patients which emerged were: the disease has been diagnosed longer ago for the volunteers and they are more inclined than patients to become angry, to try to act out their negative feelings and to try to organize their thoughts. In the breast cancer group we found that the volunteers were older than the patients, their family had a higher income and they had had a higher education; volunteers claimed to have been worse informed than patients over possibilities for information and support after their discharge from hospital.

Thus, among other things, certain coping strategies and events in the past seem to contribute to the decision to become a volunteer. A similar tendency was found in this study with respect to the adoption by patients of an unproven diet remedy (the 'Moerman' diet). We found that patients who believed they had received insufficient and unclear information from their medical specialist were more likely to adopt the Moerman diet than patients who believed the information was adequate. Personality analyses indicated also that the relationship between information adequacy and diet adoption held specifically for those patients with high trait anxiety, chronic low self-esteem, or impulsive and angry aggressive coping styles (23).

A frequently discussed topic in after-care organisations is the qualification or experience of the volunteer. For breast cancer patients, there seems to be a preference for a volunteer who has learned to cope with the problems and uncertainties of the illness and who is experienced in her volunteer work. If the more experienced volunteer is the best person to help new patients, he or she should be able to identify the patients' needs more accurately than the 'short-term' volunteer. Therefore we made a comparison between 'long-term' (doing voluntary work for more than two years) and 'short-term' (doing voluntary work for less than two years) volunteers, with respect to their activities and their estimates of new patients' needs.

With respect to their activities we found that 'short-term' volunteers engage in more face-to-face contacts and make more home visits than 'long-term' volunteers. On the other hand, 'long-term' volunteers take more part in activities involving dissemination of knowledge and representation of the patient. It seems that a shift takes place in the course of time in a volunteer's work.

With respect to the volunteers' estimation of new patients' needs it appeared that volunteers of less than two years' standing made a better appraisal of new patients' needs than did their more experienced colleagues. In general, however, volunteers' estimates of priorities in the patients' needs did not always agree with the actual needs mentioned by the patient. Breast cancer patients reported that their greatest need for information was about the origin of their disease, while vounteers estimated that this need was one of the least important. Also, volunteers estimated that the patients' most important need for information is about prostheses, while the patients themselves reported this less often. It seems that the volunteer makes a higher estimate particularly of those needs for which she can actually offer concrete information and help.

Among those who are directly involved in self-help groups, there is, in general, no doubt that such groups are useful or effective. Positive aspects mentioned include mutual support, feelings of standing together, exchange of information on physical, emotional or social consequences of treatment, emotional support and understanding and the like. By opponents and critics, however, the negative consequences or dangers of self-help groups are emphasized. Often mentioned are the inability to discriminate between different coping styles of patients, and between symptoms of the illness by which the future of the patient can be judged. False expectations could be raised and unnecessary anxiety could be evoked. Another argument of opponents is that anxiety is frequently evoked if a fellow patient dies.

We saw that an important motive for offering volunteer help is for the personal development of the volunteer. We also saw that the longer the volunteer performs volunteer work, the less accurate her estimate of the needs of new patients. From these findings it seems justified to ask the question 'how long should a volunteer do her work?' Another motive frequently mentioned by volunteers was their own unhappy experiences with the professional system. The question arises: to what

110

extent are some of the working methods of the volunteer liable to professionalisation? Finally we should ask ourselves whether criteria for the selection of new volunteers should be formulated. If so, what kind of criteria? Are the motives of new volunteers a selection criterion?

Conclusion

Help given by a volunteer is not a panacea for all patients, but a relatively large group of patients actually need this kind of support. Patients want to be informed about how other cancer patients cope with their problems. We can also conclude that for a majority of those who had contact with a fellow patient, the contact seems to be effective and beneficial.

There is still a relatively large group of patients who find it difficult to contact a volunteer. The obstacles can be inside the patient (for instance, she does not dare to phone the volunteer) or they can lie outside the patient (for instance, the physician does not tell her about the possibilities of volunteer-help). For such patients we have composed a book about possible problems and coping strategies, based on fragments of diaries of cancer patients. A patient comes to realise that he or she is not the only one who experiences specific problems and the diaries of fellow sufferers can also function as an 'eye-opener' in the selection of coping strategies.

References

1. Molleman, E., and Pruyn, J. (1981). Verwerken van kanker. Project Poliklinische Zorg Oncologie Patiënten. Studiecentrum voor Sociale Oncologie, Rotterdam.
2. Pruyn, J.F.A., (1983). Coping with stress in cancer patients; Patient education and counselling, 5, 57–62.
3. Borne, H.W. van den, Pruyn, J.F.A. (1983). Achtergronden en betekenis van lotgenotencontact bij kankerpatiënten; IVA, Tilburg.
4. Geelen, K.R.J., Pruyn, J.F.A., van den Borne, H.W., van Brunschot, C.J.M. (1984). Het verwerken van levensbedreigende ziekten: aangrijpingspunten voor patiëntenvoorlichting en ondersteuning; IVA, Tilburg.
5. Borne, H.W. van den, Pruyn, J.F.A. (1984). Informatiebehoefte en lotgenotencontact bij kankerpatiënten; Gezondheid en Samenleving, 3, 180–187
6. Lee, P.C. (1981). The psychological impact of cancer: an evaluation of laryngectomy, mastectomy and ostomy rehabilitation service programs for cancer patients; Dissertations Abstracts International, 41, 3266.
7. Logan, K., McDonald, T. (1984). Three cancer self-help groups: an exploration of their structure, process and effect on rehabilitations; Dissertations Abstracts International, 44, 2250.
8. Maisiak, R., Cain, M., Henke, C., Josof, L. (1979). An evaluation survey of TOUCH (1978) – A self-help cancer counselling program; University of Alabama in Birmingham.
9. Spiegel, D., Bloom, J.R., Yalom, I. (1981). Group support for patients with metastatic cancer – a randomized prospective outcome study; Archives of General Psychiatry, 38, 527–533.

10. Stecchi, J.H. (1979). The effects of the Reach to Recovery program on the Quality of Life and Rehabilitation of women who have had a mastectomy; Boston University.

11. Trainor, M.A. (1982). Acceptance of ostomy and the visitor role in a self-help group for ostomy patients; Nursing Research, 31, 102–106.

12. Winick, L., Robbins, G.F. (1977). Physical and psychological readjustment after mastectomy – an evaluation of Memorial Hospitals' PMRG program; Cancer, 39, 478–486.

13. Jacobs, C., Ross, R.D., Walker, I.M., Stockdale, F.E. (1983). Behavior of cancer patients: a randomized study of the effects of education and peer support groups; American Journal of Clinical Oncology, 6, 347–350.

14. Farash, J.L. (1979). Effect of counseling on resolution of loss and body image disturbance following a mastectomy; Dissertation Abstracts International, 39, 4027.

15. Vachon, M.L.S., Lyall, W.A.L., Rogers, J., Crochane, J., Freeman, S.J.J. (1981). The effectiveness of psycho-social support during post-surgical treatment of breast cancer; International Journal of Psychiatry in Medicine, 11, 365–372.

16. Hueting, S. (1980). Borstamputatie ..., daar is over te praten: In: Veranderen door onderzoek (Eds. R. de Hoog, H. Stroomberg and H. van de Zee), Boom Meppel, 253–265.

17. Steiger, M. (1981). Women's perceptions of a mastectomy self-help support-group experience; University of California, San Francisco.

18. Dam-Karskens, K. van, Nuijt-van Osnabrugge, H. (1980). Waar je mee blijft zitten als er iets wordt weggehaald – een onderzoek naar de ervaringen van vrouwen in een praatgroep na een borstamputatie. Overveen–Haarlem.

19. Heffron, W.A., Bommelaere, K., Masters, R. (1973). Group discussions with the parents of leukemic children; Pediatrics, 52, 831–840.

20. Spiegel, D., Yalom, I.D. (1978). A support group for dying patients; International Journal of Group Psychotherapy, 28, 233–245.

21. Schachter, S. (1959). The psychology of affiliation; Stanford, California, Stanford University Press.

22. Kelley, H.H. (1971). Attribution in social interaction, Morris Town, New Yersey, General Learning process.

23. Pruyn, J.F.A., Rijckman, R.M., van Brunschot, C.J.M., van den Borne, H.W..(1985). Cancer patients' personality characteristics, physician-patient communication and the adoption of the Moerman diet. Social Science and Medicine, 20, 841–847.

24. Riessman, F. (1985). The 'helper'-therapy principle; Social Work, 10, 27–32.

Chapter 12

Monitoring of Coping

MARTIN S. LEE

The monitoring of coping in the cancer patient is vital both for the patient and the family, yet it is rarely practised by clinicians. Either they find it too emotionally-threatening or time-consuming, or else they are not able to do it effectively. But coping may be monitored by a variety of clinical professionals and need not be undertaken solely by the doctor in charge of cancer treatment.

In fact, the latter always may not be the best person to monitor coping because patients may be reluctant to tell the doctor of their distress, particularly if it seems to imply criticism of the treatment. For example, a woman who has been treated for breast cancer by a breast-conserving technique may be reluctant to tell the doctor that she is distressed because the treated breast has changed in shape. Her reluctance stems from the fear that conveying her disappointment will imply criticism.

Thus, doctors, nurses, social workers, psychologists or counsellors may all be involved in monitoring the patient's ability to cope. Such clinicians need to be trained to look for the characteristics of cancer patients who fail to cope, and the evidence that they are failing to cope. Training should include instruction in interviewing techniques where the clinician learns not only what questions to ask, but also how to ask them, and how to identify non-verbal communications from the patient. In addition, professionals learning how to interview should see videotapes of their performance. Students shown their mistakes on videotape acquire better skills than those taught by conventional methods (1).

Communication failures are common (2) and an unskilled interviewer may fail to collect the desired information from the patient. Professionals need to be taught to ask open questions ("Tell me about your sleeping") as these lead to the collection of more information. Closed questions ("Do you sleep badly?") may result in the collection of inadequate or biased information. Other interviewing techniques such as facilitation and clarification (3) will also aid the interviewer. Facilitation may be verbal ("Go on, tell me more about that.") or non-verbal by for example, nodding the head. Clarification may be the asking of direct questions about the onset of symptoms and their frequency, and about the precipitating or relieving factors.

A controlled trial has examined whether monitoring by a specialist nurse can prevent the psychiatric morbidity associated with mastectomy and breast cancer (4). It found that the nurses regular monitoring led her to recognise and refer 76% of those women who needed psychiatric help. The control group received only the care normally given by the surgical unit and of this group, only 15% of those whose condition warranted help were recognised and referred.

The Concept of Coping

It is important to attempt to define what is being monitored. Coping is 'action directed at the resolution or mitigation of a problematic situation' (5), or 'the things that people do to avoid being harmed by life-strains' (6). Coping behaviour which aims at the resolution of a problem is described as a coping strategy.

Silberfarb (7) regards adaptation as a more suitable concept in the case of the cancer patient than either coping, mastery or defence. He argues that adaptation focuses on the process of adjusting to cancer as a chronic disease, while coping tends to be used more for acute and dramatic events. Mastery refers to an end point of behaviour in which 'frustations have been surmounted and adaptive efforts have come to successful conclusion.' Mastery can therefore be regarded as the proper therapeutic aim for the clinician monitoring coping in the cancer patient.

Monitoring of coping clearly involves more than a single interview with a patient. It is an ongoing process of assessment, although the initial interview with the patient is particularly important. The interviewer should try to form a warm rapport with the patient so that he feels able to share his worries and problems. A careful medical, psychiatric, family and social history should be taken and from this information, predictions about future adjustment may be made. The mental state of the patient during the interview should be noted in order to assess the current emotional adjustment. Subsequent monitoring will involve updating the history and adding information about the patient's response to the problems resulting from the illness.

An acute stress response is most commonly observed at several points in the course of the illness (8):
- At the time of diagnosis or recurrence.
- Following loss of body function or body part due to illness or treatment.
- When repeated complications occur, leading to serious limitations in functioning.
- When effective treatments have been exhausted.
- When social support fails.

Monitoring should therefore be particularly vigilant during these periods of crisis.

Evidence of Failure of Coping

The monitoring of the patient during the course of the illness involves collecting information about the patient's functioning as a whole person including the psychological, physical and social functioning. It is then assessed in relation to the type of cancer, the treatment and the prognosis. Failure of coping results in psychological distress, and it is determined whether anxiety or depression are present. The patient's view of his illness, his self concept and his future should also be inquired into and the use and abuse of psychotropic drugs and alcohol should be noted.

Many research studies have described the prevalence of psychiatric disorders in cancer patients, but there are discrepancies with regard to the frequency and nature of the disorders. A recent study carried out in the United States (9) found that 44% of 215 cancer patients manifested a psychiatric disorder. These included 68% adjustment disorders, 13% major affective disorders (depression), 8% organic mental disorders, 7% personality disorders and 4% anxiety disorders. However, other studies have suggested that only between 15 to 20% of patients are significantly depressed following the diagnosis of cancer (see Chapter 6).

In cancer patients, monitoring has most often aimed at the identification of depression and anxiety. Both conditions cause disturbances in four interacting areas: behaviour, affect (or feelings), cognition (or thoughts) and somatic (or body function). Symptoms should thus be sought from these areas. However, symptoms related to body function should be interpreted with caution in any medical patient and especially in the cancer patient. For example, loss of energy, fatigue, constipation and anorexia are symptoms of depression but may also be caused by the cancer itself or by treatment given. Check-lists used to assess anxiety or depression may therefore yield false-positive cases if they contain many items related to somatic symptoms.

Anxiety state is characterised by chronic nervousness with recurrent anxiety attacks manifested by apprehension, fearfulness or a sense of impending doom. The following symptoms may occur during attacks: shortness of breath, palpitations, chest pain or discomfort, choking sensations, dizziness and paraesthesia. Depression includes feelings of sadness, despondency, hopelessness, fearfulness, irritability and worry. Other symptoms may also be present, including poor appetite, weight loss, sleep difficulty, loss of energy, agitation or retardation, loss of interest, decrease in sexual drive, feelings of self-reproach or guilt, complaints of diminished ability to think or concentrate, and recurrent thoughts of death or suicide. It is an illness defined as lasting at least one month (10).

The patient may try to mask unpleasant feelings of hopelessness, sadness or fear by the use of tranquillisers or alcohol, but few studies report the extent of this misuse. A prevalence of only 0.5% was reported in the study by Derogatis et al (9) but this seems rather low, especially in view of the increased risk for several types of cancer in alcoholic patients. Another study found that more than a third of patients stated that their tranquilliser use increased, and 15.4% reported that their alcohol use increased, after mastectomy (11). Increasing tranquilliser use or alcohol abuse should alert the clinician to the probability that the patient is failing to cope.

Factors Related to Failure of Coping

Psychological adjustment to the disease depends partly on the patient and his or her psychosocial environment and partly on the disease, its course and treatment. Those factors derived from the patient and his environment can be further divided into pre-treatment and post-treatment factors (12).

Pre-treatment Factors

Several studies have now demonstrated psychosocial characteristics which can distinguish between patients who adjust well and those who adjust badly. The pre-treatment factors include:
- Previous psychiatric treatment.
- Evidence of depression at the time of diagnosis.
- Lack of social support or anticipated lack of support.
- Lack of employment.
- Previous personality disorder.

Weisman (13), using a scale designed to determine emotional distress, assessed the impact of diagnosis on 163 new patients in order to assess clues for later emotional distress. It was found that the more vulnerable patients had more symptoms when first diagnosed and they were generally pessimistic, anticipating little recovery and little support from other people. In addition they had more marital problems, tended to suppress feelings, and often had a history of depression. They had regrets about the past and a tendency to feel worthless. Patients of lower socioeconomic class were generally more vulnerable.

Other researchers have found that evidence of depression at the time of cancer diagnosis predicts future distress. Morris (14) studying women admitted to hospital for breast biopsy, used the Hamilton Rating Scale to measure depression. She found that women who scored 10 or more on the scale pre-operatively were significantly more likely to remain stressed by mastectomy at 2 years, whether or not they had a previous history of depressive illness. Of 42 patients who had received radiotherapy for malignant tumours, the 33 who had returned to work 9 months later showed significantly lower scores on the Depression and Morale Loss Scale of the Minnesota Multiphasic Personality Inventory and significantly higher scores on the Well Being Scale (15).

Whilst the conclusion that pre-treatment depression predicts post-treatment adjustment problems is a reasonable one, the studies quoted used different measures of depression and different outcome measures. It is not clear to what extent the measured level of depression corresponds with depression in the clinical sense.

Studies have shown that anticipated or actual lack of support characterises those individuals who fail to adjust (13, 16). Bloom (17) measured social support in breast cancer patients using measures of the cohesiveness of their family, perception of social contact, perception of amount of leisure activity and the presence of a confidant. Social support had indirect effects on all three measures of adjustment used (self-concept, sense of power and psychological distress) but these are difficult to relate to psychological states in the clinical setting.

Morris et al (14) found that none of their pre-operative psychosocial factors (including marital, sexual, interpersonal relationships and work satisfaction) clearly predicted adjustment in breast cancer patients. This study clearly shows the importance of a control group when studying the psychosocial variables, as their benign breast disease control group also had a high level of disruptions in the above psychosocial functions.

Another study of mastectomy patients found that those women reporting better emotional adjustment had been married longer, were older, and perceived significantly more understanding and emotional support from their physicians, spouses, nursing staff and children (11). Two major criticisms of the study are biased sampling and the fact that presurgery adjustment was rated several months after the operation, a method likely to lead to faulty assessment. Lack of employment seems to be a further social factor, which characterises those patients that fail to adjust (16, 17).

In summary, the role of social factors in affecting adjustment to cancer is unclear. Although one might expect their influence to be important, this is not always confirmed by research studies.

Much has been written about the importance of the patient's personality in determining their psychological response, but the common weakness of the studies has been with regard to the time of testing. The personality measures have generally been made near to the time of diagnosis (and often whilst the patient has been awaiting a surgical operation) and it is questionable whether this situation leads to valid testing of previous personality. Morris (14) found that those patients who remained stressed two years after mastectomy were characterised by high levels of neuroticism as measured on the Eysenck Personality Inventory. This finding that pre-operative neurotic traits predicts post-operative adjustment problems is borne out by other studies (11, 15, 18).

A study of women with advanced carcinoma of the cervix suggest that personality factors are associated with the perception and communication of pain (19). Patients who experienced pain and complained of it had high neuroticism and extraversion scores on the Eysenck Personalty Inventory. Those who did not perceive pain had low neuroticism and high extraversion scores, whilst those who experienced pain but did not complain had high neuroticism and low extraversion scores.

Factors during the Illness

During the course of the illness, certain psychosocial factors have been found to be related to failure of coping, and to some extent they overlap those already discussed. Thus lack of social support at the time of diagnosis or during the illness makes the patient more vulnerable.

There are many reports on the coping styles and defence mechanisms used by cancer patients. Morris et al (14) categorises five response patterns to the diagnosis of breast cancer: denial, fighting spirit, stoic acceptance, anxious or depressed acceptance, and an attitude of hopelessness and helplessness. Interestingly, those patients displaying denial or fighting spirit were subsequently shown to have a significantly better outlook in terms of recurrence-free survival at 5 years. Katz et al (20) similarly describe six defence styles: displacement, projection, denial, stoicism/fatalism, prayer/faith and mixed. Using ratings of disruption in life function, unpleasant affect and indices of adrenocortical function as measures of psychological and physiological disturbance, they found denial, stoicism, and prayer to be the most successful means of coping.

Weisman (13) described four vulnerability factors derived by factor analysis and these he named denial, annihilation, alienation and destructive dysphoria. He found that more vulnerable patients tended to vacillate between denial and acceptance. Ray et al (5) studying mastectomy and hernia patients, have suggested six coping 'themes' in respect to the patients' orientation to the threat. The themes of rejection, control, resignation, minimisation, avoidance and dependency are not mutually exclusive so that a patient may have a 'repertoire' of themes. Recently, attempts have been made to devise a method for rating cognitive responses to a diagnosis of cancer (21).

Changes in self esteem are an important reaction in cancer patients. Self esteem is related to body image, performance, and quality of interpersonal relations, and all of these may be threatened by the diagnosis of cancer. Mutilating operations such as mastectomy, colostomy and amputation are likely to affect the feelings and thoughts experienced in relation to one's body (see Chapter 3). Cancer patients may have difficulty in performing everyday activities and changes in their work performance, hobbies and leisure activities may result in their feeling less needed, and so affect their self esteem. Changes in self esteem may lead to depression, and the feelings of worthlessness associated with depression may then further reduce self esteem. Questions aimed at determining a patient's self esteem are particularly important in the assessment of coping.

Factors Related to the Disease and its Treatment

It is impossible to separate the emotional response to the disease itself from response to the effects of treatment. Symptoms from the disease may increase the likelihood of failure of coping and these need to be noted during monitoring. Weisman (13), studying patients with cancers of the breast, lung, colon, Hodgkin's disease and malignant melanoma found that the anatomical type of cancer did not relate to the level of vulnerability. However, more severe somatic symptoms were found to relate to current and future distress, and those presenting at an advanced stage usually had more symptoms.

Psychological distress in patients undergoing surgery is discussed in Chapter 3. Devlin et al (22) found that depression, social isolation and particularly sexual problems were common in patients treated by abdominoperineal resection and colostomy for anorectal tumours. Depression and isolation have been described following disfiguring surgery for maxillo-facial cancer. Wochnik (23) in a questionnaire survey found that four years after laryngectomy, approximately 50% of patients suffered from a depressive state which impaired work capacity and personal relationships.

Multiple physical treatments should alert the clinician to the increased likelihood of failure of coping. Adding one year of chemotherapy to surgery and radiotherapy for breast cancer has been shown to produce significantly greater depression at 18 months later than radiotherapy alone (24). Similarly, Maguire (25) found a high incidence of psychiatric morbidity in patients given adjuvant chemotherapy and suggested that it was linked to symptoms of physical toxicity.

Caring for cancer in the young is discussed in Chapter 15 but it must be stressed that to monitor the child's ability to cope it is necessary to monitor the whole family. The effect of a cancer in childhood has a marked effect on the parents and a study of children dying from leukaemia showed that in half the families, at least one member reacted so intensely as to need psychiatric treatment for the first time (26). Friedman et al (27) described the parents' response as shock followed by hostility, anger and anticipatory grief. The child's illness results in strain on the parents' marriage and it has been reported that a quarter of marriages break down under the stress.

Monitoring coping in children will involve not only observing the child's emotional reactions and those of the family but also the communications between them. An often crucial communication is what the parents disclose to the child about the diagnosis. Binger et al (26) suggest that the children who appeared most lonely were those who were aware of the diagnosis, but whose parents did not wish them to know. Coping with the illness may therefore be aided by disclosure of the diagnosis in such circumstances.

Monitoring coping and managing treatment in the child and family is a stressful task. The clinicians themselves may be the target of anger and hostility, and may themselves find it difficult to cope.

120

Conclusion

In order to monitor coping, the clinician requires adequate knowledge and sensitivity, and particular skills are required in interviewing techniques. A plan should be made to enable the monitoring of the patient alongside treatment reviews and the clinician needs to be aware of the times during the illness when the stresses are greatest and what to look for in order to monitor failure of coping.

Psychological adjustment depends partly on the patient and his or her psychosocial environment, and partly on medical factors related to the illness and treatment. Pre-treatment factors have been identified which predict a greater likelihood of failure of coping. During the illness the patient may use various coping themes or styles and may vacillate between them.

Whilst some patients show failure to cope with their illness, a large percentage appear to successfully adapt to the streses imposed upon them. The aim of monitoring coping is to identify those patients who are experiencing difficulties, and help them achieve a quality of life that is acceptable to them.

References

1. Maguire, G.P., Goldberg, D., Jones, S., Hyde, C., O'Down, T. (1978). The value of feedback in teaching interviewing skills to medical students. Psychological Medicine, 8, 695–704.
2. Fletcher, C. 1980. Listening and talking to patients. I. British Medical Journal, 281, 845–847.
3. Fletcher, c. (1980). Listening and talking to patients. II. British Medical Journal, 281, 931–933.
4. Maguire, P., Tait, A., Brooke, M., Thomas, C., Sellwood, R. (1980). Effect of counselling on the psychiatric morbidity associated with mastectomy. British Medical Journal, 281, 1454–1456.
5. Ray, C., Lindop, J., Gibson, S. (1982). The concept of coping. Psychological Medicine, 12, 385–395.
6. Pearlin, L., Schooler, C. (1978). The structure of coping. Journal of Health and Social Behaviour, 19, 2–21.
7. Silberfarb, P.M. (1982). Research in adaptation to illness and psychosocial intervention. Cancer, 50, 1921–1925.
8. Gorzynski, J.G. (1982). Depression in cancer patients: prevalence, diagnosis and psychotropic drug management. Current Concepts in Psychosocial Oncology, Memorial Sloan-Kettering Cancer Centre, New York, p. 23.
9. Derogatis, L.R., Morrow, G.R., Fetting, J., Penman, D., Piasetsky, S., Schmale, A.M., Henrichs, M., Carnicke, C.L.M. (1983). The prevalence of psychiatric disorders among cancer patients. Journal of the American Medical Association, 249, 751–757.
10. Feighner, J.P., Robins, E., Guze, S.B., Woodruff, R.A., Winokur, G., Munoz, (1972). Diagnostic criteria for use in psychiatric research. Archives of General Psychiatry, 26, 57–63.
11. Jamison, K.R., Wellisch, D.K., Pasnau, R.O. (1978). Psychosocial aspects of mastectomy: I. The woman's perspective. American Journal of Psychiatry, 135;; 432–436.
12. Holland, J.C., Mastrovito, R. (1980). Psychologic adaptation to breast cancer. Cancer, 46, 1045–1052.
13. Weisman, A.D. (1976). Early diagnosis of vulnerability in cancer patients. American Journal of the Medical Sciences, 271, 187–196.

14. Morris, B.A., Greer, H.S., White, P. (1977). Psychological and social adjustment to mastectomy. Cancer, 40, 2381–2387.
15. Schonfield, J. (1972). Psychological factors related to a delayed return to an earleir life-style in successfully treated cancer patients. Journal of Psychosomatic Research, 16, 41–46.
16. Coblimer, W.G. (1977) Psychosocial factors in gynaecological or breast malignancies. Hospital Physician, 10, 38–40.
17. Bloom, J.R. (1982). Social support, accomodation to stress and adjustment to breast cancer. Social Science and Medicine, 16, 1329–1338.
18. Hughes, J. (1982). Emotional reactions to the diagnosis and treatment of early breast cancer. Journal of Psychosomatic Research, 26, 277–283.
19. Bond, M.R. *1971). The relation of pain to the Eysenck personality Inventory, Cornell Medical Index and Whiteley Index of Hypochondriasis. British Journal of Psychiatry, 119, 641–678.
20. Katz, J.L., Weiner, H., Gallagher, T.F., Hellman, L. (1970). Stress distress and ego defences: Psychoendocrine response to impending breast tumour biopsy. Archives of General Psychiatry, 23, 131–142.
21. Morris, T., Blake, S., Buckley, M. (1985). Development of a method for rating cognitive responses to a diganosis of cancer. Social Science and Medicine (in press).
22. Devlin, H.B., Plant, J.A., Griffin, M. (1971). Aftermath of surgery for anorectal cancer. British Medical Journal, 3, 413–418.
23. Wochnik, M. (1976). Psychologische Erhebungen bei Kehlkopfexterpierten. Zeitschrift für ärtztliche Fortbildung, 70, 1213–1218.
24. Cooper, A.F., McArdle, C.S., Russel, A.R., Smith, D.C. (1979). Psychiatric morbidity associated with adjuvant chemotherapy following mastectomy for breast cancer. British Journal of Surgery, 66, 362.
25. Maguire, G.P., Tait, A., Brooke, M., Thomas, C., Howat, J.M.T., Sellwood, R.A., Bush, H. (1980). Psychiatric morbidity and physical toxicity associated with adjuvant chemotherapy after mastectomy. British Medical Journal, 281, 1179–1180.
26. Binger, C.M., Ablin, A.R., Feurstein, R.C., Kushner, J.H., Zoger, S., Mikkelsen, C. (1969). Childhood leukaemia: emotional impact on patient and family. New England Journal of Medicine, 280, 414–418.
27. Friedman, S.B., Chodoff, P., Mason, J.W., Hamburg, D.A. (1963). Behavioural observations on parents anticipating the death of a child. Paediatrics, 32, 610–625.

Chapter 13

Results of Supportive Therapy

MAGGIE WATSON

It is clear that the emotional cost of cancer is high (1, 2) and many have begun to ask whether the distress associated with the diagnosis and treatment can be alleviated by specific supportive therapies. Two practical questions arise – to whom should support be directed and what is the most effective method? The former question was discussed in the previous chapter.

A recent review (3) concluded that the evidence of benefit from supportive therapy is equivocal and that the advantages of one type of support over another remain unproven. This is not because of a lack of support programmes, but a dearth of well controlled studies evaluating the many programmes. This makes it difficult to draw conclusions as to which methods produce benefit.

An equally important problem in evaluating supportive therapy is inadequate description of the therapeutic methods used. Reports often lack sufficient depth and clarity to allow another clinician to repeat a particular programme. The studies included in this review meet the following criteria: a description of the type of support offered; a control group included in the evaluation; sufficient statistical analysis included to allow the reader to derive a conclusion.

It is useful to consider early and late stage cancer patients as two different groups, as their problems are greatly influenced by the stage of their disease. They often represent quite different therapeutic groups when it comes to considering their needs.

Studies with Early Stage Patients

Bloom's group (4) have described an individual counselling programme for mastectomy patients which included a Reach-to-Recovery visitor to provide a successful role model, and an oncology counsellor to provide support and information during the period of the patient's hospital stay. After discharge from hospital, a social worker provided co-ordination and continuity of the service between the hospital and community.

No significant changes in mood state were found when measured two months post-operatively, but nevertheless this programme served to increase feelings of control when these were measured using a health locus-of-control scale. The importance of such feelings in aiding adjustment were emphasized by the authors. They were also of the opinion that the oncology counsellor should be part of the surgical, rather than the nursing, psychiatric or social services staff, to ensure close co-ordination with the medical team.

A more recent study (5) described the results of an individual counselling service for mastectomy patients, which was offered by a specialist nurse who was a member of the surgical staff. Although information about physical state and prosthetic advice was offered, the main therapeutic component involved emotional support and facilitation of adjustment through counselling. The overall aim was to give the patient an opportunity to express feelings, discuss problems and explore any anxieties. Discussions were not confined to problems arising from the diagnosis and treatment, but other problems hindering adjustment were included. The patient was encouraged to draw on her own resources when trying to adjust. If she responded inappropriately, she was guided toward more constructive methods of coping. Psychiatric referrals were made when severe reactions occurred, and where necessary, patients were referred to other agencies for specialist advice.

Results from an evaluation of this service were encouraging. Counselled patients appeared to make a more rapid adjustment than those receiving routine care. The overall effect of counselling on mood, particularly depression, appears to have been to encourage a more rapid decrease in negative affect and greater feelings of personal control. Family members were included in this service and this appears to have encouraged discussion between the patient and spouse, with a tendency among counselled patients to confide more in their spouse and family.

Both this study and the study by Bloom and colleagues, highlight the need for counselling to continue beyond the immediate pre- and post-operative period. In both studies no clear benefits were found during the week or two following surgery. Some two to three months post-operatively, however, the benefits of counselling appeared to have accrued. Despite the lack of short term benefit, counselling during the early period, particularly pre-operatively, seemed crucial in establishing a knowledgeable and trusting bond between counsellor and patient, and provided the foundation for their continuing relationship. These results emphasize the need for supportive therapy to extend beyond the initial period of diagnosis and primary treatment and to be available as the need arises, with patients being reviewed at follow-up clinics. It would also appear that in some cases responses to the stress of cancer may only be changed through protracted therapeutic intervention.

Counselling, as a therapeutic method, seems particularly well-suited to the majority of early stage patients who, by and large, are 'normal people' suffering a severe and acute stress. There is some indication that the counselling approach is effective in shifting transient mood state but may be less effective in changing entrenched behavioural responses and more severe disturbance. It may be, that for the majority of early stage cancer patients, a programme of counselling is adequate for their needs. However, more research is needed to confirm these findings and there is also a need to determine more clearly which components of counselling have the most therapeutic value.

Capone's group (6) have described a rehabilitation service for gynaecological cancer patients. This too was an individual counselling programme specifically modelled on a crisis intervention approach. Patients were counselled on a minimum of four occasions during their hospital stay, with at least one session prior to primary treatment and the last session just before discharge from hospital. The types of problem dealt with, the number of sessions and the length of sessions, were all tailored by the therapist to individual needs.

In general, early sessions were directed toward helping patients express feelings of concern, anger and guilt, and fear related to treatment or death. Self-esteem and femininity were the focus of the middle sessions, whilst the final sessions focussed on interpersonal relationships with family and others. For sexually active patients, the problems of sexual rehabilitation were also addressed. (In this group of patients sexual problems are known to be common because of the nature of their cancer.) Although the authors could show no clear benefits in terms of improved mood state, the counselled patients reported a clear and more positive self-image, and more of them had returned to work and to their pre-morbid level of sexual functioning than had the non-counselled group, when these variables were measured at a 12 month follow-up.

Another study (7) compared mastectomy patients who received 12 weekly sessions of crisis counselling, with a second group who had participated over the same period in a self-help counselling group. The level of depression reported was not significantly different, compared to a control group, although the control group did show more body image disturbance than either of the two therapy groups. There was no evidence that one therapeutic method had any advantage over the other, although both had advantages over no therapy at all.

The programme evolved by Gordon and his colleagues (8) begins with an overall treatment plan covering three different areas: 1. Educating the patient about how to live with the disease effectively, including providing information about the medical system and the patient's condition. 2. Counselling which focussed on reactions and feelings about the disease, with the patient being encouraged to ventilate feelings. 3. An area which they called 'environmental' and including formal service referrals to appropriate agencies and other health care personnel.

However, the nature and extent of the intervention varied for each patient so that individual therapy plans were developed and revised as appropriate. The frequency and duration of this supportive therapy was not limited on any *a priori* basis. As a result of this programme of supportive therapy, negative affect declined more rapidly after the patients were discharged from hospital. Six months after discharge, this group reported a more realistic outlook on life and a greater number had returned to work.

As patients with a variety of cancers were included in the study, it was possible to make some evaluation of their differing needs. It was found, that each cancer site had associated with it different clinical issues, with different patterns of psychological recovery and negative effect. Gordon's group concluded that the actual supportive method, although perhaps following a general framework, will depend to a great extent on cancer site and stage.

Jacobs and colleagues (9) set up a study to determine whether a programme of patient education would be more, or less, effective in enhancing psychological function, in a group of patients with Hodgkin's disease, than a peer support therapy group. In the educational arm of this trial each patient received a 27-page booklet about Hodgkin's disease, in which was discussed diagnosis, staging, treatment methods, treatment problems and prognosis. Patients also received newsletters which contained information on recent advances in the treatment of Hodgkin's disease. For the peer support group the main thrust of therapy was the attendance at weekly meetings over a period of eight weeks where the aim was to stimulate discussions about issues of concern to these patients. The groups were attended by an oncologist, psychologist and social worker, in non-directive roles.

At the end of the educational intervention, both anxiety- and treatment-related problems were reduced in this group when compared to a control group. For the peer support group an improvement in depression and anxiety was observed but this was also found to the same extent in the control group, with no additional benefits appearing to be derived from participation in supportive group therapy. The authors observed, when trying to explain the benefits derived from the educational programme and the lack of benefit from the group therapy programme, that the effectiveness of education may have been influenced by the type of cancer. It seems likely that, in a cancer which has a good possibility of cure, an educational programme might be more effective. They went on to say that 'it may be that peer support groups did not alter the behavior of patients with a potentially curable disease such as Hodgkin's disease.'

The main goals of the supportive therapies described above were the reduction of psychological morbidity, in particular a decrease in anxiety and depression, and the enhancement of positive attitudes. Other chapters in this book discuss the effectiveness of therapy designed to promote sexual rehabilitation and the use of relaxation and desensitization procedures in the treatment of the conditioned nausea experienced by some patients in protracted chemotherapy.

Studies with Late Stage Patients

In one study (10) supportive therapy was extended to a small group of adults with newly diagnosed metastasis. Supportive therapy offered to these patients was based on a crisis intervention model, with a strong educational emphasis. The basic assumption underlying this programme, was that the more patients knew about the varying aspects of their disease, the more they would be able to handle their problems. For patients who do not appear to use denial as a defence against the emotional impact of cancer, it is probably true that information intended to demystify the disease and its treatment, may assist their understanding and thereby return to them some feelings of control. Such programmes may do the important job of dispelling the more frightening myths surrounding cancer. In this study the support group met on six occasions at the rate of three sessions a week.

As a result of this therapy the patients reported greater confidence in the medical staff and a better understanding of the various aspects of cancer. They were also considered more at ease with their reactions and feelings about death. What was not clear, however, was the extent to which emotional distress was alleviated by this programme. The authors appear to interpret these positive attitudes as evidence of adjustment and, therefore, presumably less distress.

Controlled studies in which death counselling has been evaluated, are rare, although it is quite common for patients in the terminal phase of their illness to receive some counselling or support. One study (11), as reported in Chapter 17, appears to have obtained some degree of success. The counselled group, when compared to a control group, showed improved quality of life when this was measured after 3 months in this programme. Depression was decreased when this was measured 3 months after the initiation of counselling. However, this appears to have reached an optimal level after 3 months of counselling and improvements in mood did not occur thereafter.

Group therapy also has been used to support dying patients. Spiegel's group (12) described a series of weekly support groups which focussed on discussions of death and dying, related family problems, difficulties in obtaining treatment, and issues of communication with physicians. Unlike the usual psychotherapy group there were few process interpretations, with the participants being encouraged to live as richly as possible in the face of a terminal illness. They report that, "The fact that the members could tangibly be of help to one another reinforced their sense of still being alive and effective in the world. In fact, being of help to others, even at the very end of life, helped to imbue members with a vital sense of meaningfulness." As a result of participation in this group therapy the patients, when compared to the control group, were found to be less anxious and to use fewer maladaptive methods of managing stress. They showed a significant decrease in mood disturbance but no differences were found between the support and control groups in measures of self esteem, denial or perceptions of control over health.

More recently, these authors have examined the benefits of self-hypnosis and group therapy in women with metastatic breast cancer (13). In addition to the group therapy described in their early study, one of the two groups also ended their group session with a self-hypnosis exercise led by a psychiatrist. This was designed to help the patients alter their experience of pain. These exercises lasted for five to ten minutes and included instructions for use outside of the group. These exercises involved, 'teaching patients not to fight the pain but to "filter the hurt out of the pain" by imagining competing sensations in the affected areas, such as icy, cold numbness, or a warm tingling sensation.' In this way they were taught to change their experience of pain by focussing on competing sensations.

Pain frequency and duration were not altered by this method but the self-hypnosis group reported better control over the sensation of pain when this occurred and, whereas the control group showed a deterioration in relation to pain, those in the hypnosis group showed no increase in pain over the year following the initiation of this therapy. Interestingly, those patients included in the support group who did not receive self-hypnosis training, also reported less pain than the control group. The authors considered that the mitigation of anxiety, depression, and fatigue, associated with group support, helped these patients to experience diminished pain. These findings highlight the difficulty of determining the extent to which cancer pain might be exacerbated by anxiety or ameliorated by supportive therapy. It suggested, however, that support which combined specific pain control procedures, as well as teaching coping strategies in general, may mitigate pain for some patients. This area clearly merits further investigation.

Conclusion

It is difficult to draw conclusions from the literature on the efficacy of supportive therapy in cancer patients. There is clearly a need for more research to determine which methods are best for which patients at whatever stage of their disesae. It is possible, however, to discern some trends in terms of what seems to work and what constitute guidelines for the selection of an effective overall approach, and these are summarized as follows:

1. Adequate information given to demystify the cancer treatment and dispel the myths surrounding the illness.
2. Support which is available from the time of diagnosis.
3. The same therapist seeing the patient throughout, thereby facilitating an effective relationship.
4. Support tailored to individual needs and not limited, on *a priori* grounds, to any particular periods of time.
5. Support which directs attention to all problems hindering adjustment and not just to cancer.
6. Recognition that families play an important role and, hence, the inclusion of a family member in therapy where appropriate.

7. Therapy aimed at enhancing feelings of control and reducing feelings of helplessness.

References

1. Morris, T. (1979). Psychological adjustment to mastectomy. Cancer Treatment Reviews, 6, 41–61.
2. Meyerowitz, B.E. (1980). Psychosocial correlates of breast cancer and its treatments. Psychological Bulletin, 87, 108–131.
3. Watson, M. (1983). Psychosocial intervention with cancer patients: a review. Psychological Medicine, 13, 839–846.
4. Bloom, J.R., Ross, R.D., Burnell, G. (1978). The effect of social support on patient adjustment after breast surgery. Patient Counselling and Health Education, Autumn, 50–59.
5. Watson, M., Buckley, M., Denton, S., Blake, S., Greer, S., Baum, M. (1985). The effectiveness of a specialist nurse counselling service for mastectomy patients. Submitted for publication.
6. Capone, M.A., Good, R.S., Westie, S., Jacobson, A.F. (1980). Psychosocial rehabilitation of gynecologic oncology patients. Archives of Physical Medicine and Rehabilitation, 61, 128–132.
7. Farash, J.L. (1979). Effect of counselling on resolution of loss and body image disturbance following a mastectomy. Dissertation Abstracts International 38, 4027.
8. Gordon, W.A., Freidenbergs, I., Diller, L., Hibbard, M., Wolf, C., Levine, L., Lipkins, R., Ezrachi, O., Lucido, D. (1980). Efficacy of psychosocial intervention with cancer patients. Journal of Consulting and Clinical Psychology, 48, 743–759.
9. Jacobs, C., Ross, R.D., Walker, I.M., Stockdale, F.E. (1983). Behavior of cancer patients: a randomized study of the effects of education and peer support groups. American Journal of Clinical Oncology, 6, 347–350.
10. Ferlic, M., Goldman, A., Kennedy, B.J. (1979). Group counselling in adult patients with advanced cancer. Cancer, 43, 760–766.
11. Linn, M.W., Linn, B.S., Harris, R. (1982). Effects of counselling for late stage cancer patients. Cancer, 49, 1048–1055.
12. Spiegel, D., Bloom, J.R., Yalom, I. (1981). Group support for patients with metastatic cancer. Archives of General Psychiatry, 38, 527–533.
13. Spiegel, D., Bloom, J.R. (1983). Group therapy and hypnosis reduce metastatic breast carcinoma pain. Psychsomatic Medicine, 45, 333–339.

Chapter 14

Psychological Self-Help by Cancer Patients

ALASTAIR J. CUNNINGHAM

An important resource in fighting against cancer may be the ability many people have to learn mental techniques for helping themselves. "Self-help" is a description sometimes reserved for mutual aid groups, while "self-care" is applied to ways of coping learned from professionals or initiated and performed alone (1). However, self-help broadly includes any activity which a person learns from others or develops himself, and then maintains through his own efforts as a means of counteracting the physical or psychological effects of disease.

Unorthodox and unproven remedies in cancer fall into two main categories: dietary (or nutritional) and psychological. In a recent survey in the USA (2), the three most common unorthodox treatments used by the patients studied were "metabolic therapy," diet and megavitamins – all basically nutritional remedies; the next two most popular modalities (about half as common as the first group) were the psychological approaches of imagery and spiritual or faith healing. A mixed group of unorthodox remedies included procedures such as the injection of "immune" serum, used by about 15% of the patients.

Dietary Self-Help

Dietary change, the major mode of self-help for cancer patients, is advocated by a large, anecdotal, and often dogmatic popular literature. This is extremely confusing to patients, since the recommendations are often contradictory and vary between countries; for example birch-ash heads the list in Finland (3), while vitamin C and laetrile have displaced earlier favourites and are now the leading popular remedies in North America.

Recent reviews (4, 5) estimate that diet may contribute to human cancer in between 30% and 70% of cases. The evidence suggesting the possibility of prevention of cancer by diet (together with some inconclusive data on the role of trace minerals), has been illogically applied to its recommendation for cure – an entirely different scientific problem. There has been little scientific investigation of the purported curative effects of most nutritional aids, although controlled experiments have failed completely to show benefits from laetrile (6) or from Vitamin C (7, 8).

Dangers arising from reliance on dietary manipulation include the following (9): the risk that conventional therapy will be abandoned; possible toxicity of agents such as high doses of certain vitamins; wasting money; and finally the despair that ensues if and when the remedies fail to cure. However, to redress the balance a little, an element that seems common to all the varied nutritional therapies is their placebo effect, sense of control or source of hope.

Recommended dietary regimes, which are usually low in fat and meat protein and high in fresh vegetables and grain content, may also have other advantages over the conventional North American way of eating. In some cases, greater attention to diet may bring about an improvement in a person's eating habits and a general benefit to health. Provided conventional medical care is not abandoned, and essential nutritional elements adequately obtained, it seems unreasonable for clinicians to dismiss out of hand the self-help that many patients seek through such a diet (10, 11).

Specific Mental Self-Help Approaches

There are three possible aims for psychological intervention in the treatment of cancer. In order of increasing unconventionality they are: (1) Relief of emotional anguish and increased sense of peace and meaning. This covers the usual objective of support as discussed in the preceding chapters. (2) Increasing physical comfort in coping with medical treatment. (3) Increasing survival time or remission of disease.

Emotional support is usually taken to mean comforting, sharing of burdens, strengthening, and maintenance of emotional balance (12, 13) but does not include procedures designed primarily to change attitudes or enhance self-understanding. Its methods and results are discussed in other chapters. Professional help is provided on a one-to-one basis by counsellors, but there is a growing literature on support groups for cancer patients (14–16). Some of these are professionally led (17, 18, 19) and may be educational as well as supportive (20, 21). Others offer "self-help" in the sense of mutual patient aid (22–25). Several groups have become enormous organisations, affecting thousands of people including Reach to Recovery (26), Make Today Count (27) and others (14). Group support is not usually integrated into the general medical care of the patient, although there are exceptions to this (28–31).

Coping with Disease Symptoms and Treatment Side Effects

Such help has, as its major goal, the modification of maladaptive behaviour and thoughts, rather than the uncovering of deep-seated psychological conflict (32–34). It is concerned with helping patients alleviate such problems as nausea and vomiting, pain, anorexia, general stress and non-compliance with medical treatment.

Several studies clearly show that self-hypnosis training, progressive muscle relaxation, and systematic desensitation can all reduce the extent of the nausea and vomiting that may accompany many chemotherapeutic regimes (35, 36). The anticipatory nausea which affects about 25% of such patients (i.e. nausea before actual treatment) has been most studied and seems most susceptible to psychological change, but certain patients can learn a degree of control over the post-chemotherapy effects as well. For some individuals, the presence of a therapist is needed for best effects, while others can learn these self-control techniques for use alone, either in hospital or at home (36).

Behavioural methods such as relaxation, biofeedback and behaviour modification (37) and especially hypnosis (38–41) have proved useful adjuncts to drugs in the management of cancer pain. Self-hypnosis using imagery was found valuable for alleviation of pain and nausea in children with cancer (42), while others employed a behavioural "package" – filmed modelling, reinforcement, breathing exercises, emotive imagery and behavioural rehearsal – to help children cope with repeated painful procedures (43).

One trial (44) showed that pain and suffering were diminished when training in self-hypnosis was added to a group support programme for cancer patients. At present, pain in cancer patients is largely managed by drugs, but a case can be made for using behavioural adjunctive techniques which have shown their usefulness in other areas of pain control. Relaxation training, systematic desensitisation to reduce pain of medical procedures, hypnosis, and some cognitive procedures are now gaining acceptance in treatment of chronic pain generally (45).

The anorexia and conditioned food aversion that often accompany cancer and its treatment are problems for which behavioural intervention seems appropriate and should be further investigated (14, 33). Learned aversion to foods might be controlled by altering meal patterns and settings in cases where increased intake of food is important to the health of the patient.

Stress control (46) will not be reviewed here but various kinds of relaxation, meditation, biofeedback, hypnosis and cognitive restructuring (thought-changing) techniques have been used to combat stress, either in sessions with a therapist or learned as techniques for home use. Self-hypnosis can control insomnia and headaches as well as other pain (34), and patients can be given relaxation audiotapes for use during painful treatment procedures; this is a self-help technique which could be employed by people who have difficulty with the relaxation/self-control procedures.

Table 1. Some "self-help" techniques, relevant to improving health, that can be learned by cancer patients*

Major "level" of impact	
Spiritual/existential	Meditation (various kinds)
	Religious studies and practices (where acceptable)
Whole earth environment	Nature awareness/study
Social/cultural	Seeking support and communication with others
	Alstruistic action
Integrated body-mind	Relaxation (various kinds)
	Yoga, T'ai Chi, dance and various other ancient and modern body-awareness techniques.
	Biofeedback
Unconscious mind	Mental imagery
	Self hypnosis
	Dream recording and analysis
	Music, art.
Conscious mind	Positive affirmations
	Goal setting
	Appropriate reading
	Diary keeping for self-awareness
	Problem solving
	Assertiveness Training
	Thought-stopping
Body	Healthy life-style changes (diet, rest, recreation, physical exercise)

* Not all are appropriate for all patients, of course. Some activities could be classified in several levels.

Problem-solving approaches have been taught to cancer patients for subsequent use alone (47, 48). Exploration of "psychomotor" therapies, art, dance, Gestalt and other intense feeling modes, is advocated as a means of promoting expression of such emotions as anger or guilt (13). Many stress-relieving and awareness-promoting exercises that can be done alone might be added to this category (see Table 1) e.g. T'ai Chi, yoga, bioenergetics and other ancient and modern body-centered therapies.

Attempts to Affect the Physical Disease

There is little evidence for any clinical effect of diet on cancer growth, and no scientific rationale has been offered for effects of nutritional elements on progress of the disease (with the possible exception of vitamin C (49). However, the basis for a psychological effect is stronger (50). Evidence for mind-body effects comes from such areas as the placebo effect (51), biofeedback (52) hypnosis research (53) and psychological conditioning, for example, of immune responses (54). The argument for a mind-cancer link lies in the convergence of evidence from three separate areas of research: animal experiments, human personality studies and clinical trials. Only the last of these will be considered here.

The Simontons and their colleagues are the group most responsible for popularizing the recent application to cancer treatment of psychological techniques, particularly suggestion by mental imagery (55). Their colleagues have described a correlation between imagery on projective testing and delay in progress of the disease (56) and have developed a test, IMAGE-CA, in which patients were asked to draw pictures of their cancer, their body's defenses (especially white blood cells) and their medical treatment. After an interview, each patient's images were scored on 14 dimensions, including vividness, activity and strength of the cancer cells and the white blood cells, the patient's perception of the effectiveness of his or her defenses and treatment, and a clinician's impression of the imagery. The 14 dimensions were weighted and summed to produce a single predictive index.

Achterberg and Lawlis (56) presented some reliability data (inter-rater and interdimensional correlation) and tested the validity of the index on a sample of 58 people with advanced cancer. All patients with a score of more than 0.58 standard deviations below the mean showed new cancer or died, while almost all those scoring more than approximately 1 standard deviation above the mean showed regression of tumors or no disease.

The Simontons have taken this approach a step further, advising patients to imagine during daily relaxation periods, their defense systems as strong, their cancer cells as weak, and their medical treatment as beneficial. The imagery chosen by patients was sometimes quasi-realistic (for example, white blood cells engulfing cancer cells) and sometimes symbolic (for example, large dogs eating up piles of meat). Personal responsibility for health, the development of goals, and other lifestyle adjustments were also stressed (55).

They have reported that the median survival time of a large group of patients taking part in a programme using these approaches (in conjunction with regular medical treatment) was about twice that of people with similar diseases at several major United States treatment centers (57). These results must however be regarded as preliminary, since, as the authors themselves point out, their highly selected sample consisted of motivated, well-educated individuals who might have performed better than average without the psychotherapy. Controlled trials are needed to establish the efficacy of the approach.

A programme closely related to the Simontons', although with more emphasis on hypnosis, has recently been described by Newton (58). Patients were seen by psychologists once a week for treatments by hypnosis, visualization techniques, and general psychotherapy. Audiotapes enabled the patients to practise at home. In 8 years of work with 283 patients, 105 had 10 or more 1 hour sessions within 3 months ("adequately treated"), 57 had 3 to 9 sessions ("inadequately treated"), and the rest had less than 3 sessions. Of those adequately treated, 54 percent were alive at the time the report was written, compared with only 18 percent of the inadequately treated. This was said to be a significant difference but the study provided no analysis. Median survival times of (all?) treated patients were claimed to be 2 1/2 to 4 times the national medians (the proportions differing for different cancer sites). The study claimed that quality of life was almost universally improved, but supplied no data on this point.

While the effects reported here are impressively large, it is difficult to exclude selection bias without randomisation or stricter control procedures. For example, it may be that patients dropped out of treatment (and were therefore classified as "inadequately treated") because they had more serious illness, although the two groups were said to show no significant differences in medical status.

A third major published clinical study is by Meares (59, 60), an Australian psychiatrist who uses intensive daily meditation as the basis for his treatment of cancer patients. Of the 73 patients treated, 5 are said to have made "what appears to have been a complete regression of their growth in the absence of any organic treatment which could possibly account for it." Five others appeared to be "well on the way to similar regression" and many more apparently enjoyed significant psychological benefits.

Again, in the absence of controls and of details about the medical condition of the patients (most were said to have advanced disease), it is difficult to assess this work. It differs from the Simonton and Newton approaches in being much less directive, relying perhaps on producing a shift in the patient's perceived relationship to the world through long periods in the meditative state. Nonetheless, the reported results point in the same direction.

The three trials discussed above relied mainly on teaching techniques for patients to use in their own time, but were uncontrolled. A randomised controlled trial has recently been described (61) which also claims prolongation of life in a large number of patients as a result of psychotherapy, although in this case the intervention consisted of 20–30 hours of individual therapy. The treatment was called "creative novation", a cognitive behavioural approach in which patients were helped to express previously inhibited needs, and find new solutions to emotional problems. Relaxation and suggestion were used in addition to counselling.

This therapy was compared, in two experiments on patients with metastatic breast cancer, against more traditional behaviour modification, psychoanalytic therapy, or none. Creative novation is claimed to have increased average life span by 6–9 months. Behaviour modification, or treatment by relatively less experienced creative novation therapists, had less, but still positive effects, while the analytic psychotherapy had no effect in one experiment and shortened patients' lives by an average of 14 months in the other.

A recent, controlled study of a programme similar to those of the Simontons, Newton and Meares has shown some of the difficulties in the evaluation of these approaches (62). The Exceptional Cancer Patient (ECaP) program in New Haven has taught meditation and mental imagery to patients, and facilitated discussion of their problems, for several years. When 34 of its participants with breast cancer were individually matched on several prognostic factors, each with 3 control women who did not attend the programme, it at first appeared that average survival of the group members was significantly prolonged. However, the effect was found to be largely due to a selection bias caused by a shorter interval between cancer diagnosis and entry to the programme. Correcting for this bias removed the survival benefit, although the program participants enjoyed an improved quality of life.

Thus, we have three claims for enhanced survival based on uncontrolled trials, and two controlled studies, one claiming an increased life-span attributed to cognitive behavioural therapy, and one failing to show a survival advantage from a self-help programme. In addition, there are a number of case-reports of psychotherapy of various kinds apparently contributing to tumour regression (63–65). The case is far from proven and clearly requires further controlled trials.

The Toronto Experience

We have been conducting "Cancer Self Help" groups at a cancer hospital in Toronto, Canada for about 3 years, during which time approximately 130 people (at the time of writing) have attended a structured course consisting usually of seven 1 1/2 hour sessions per week. The course teaches most of what the literature has indicated is useful: two kinds of relaxation (progressive muscle and self-hypnotic), meditation, use of positive mental imagery and cognitive self-help techniques such as stress awareness and control, efficient time use, goal definition, thought-stopping and lifestyle planning. Attndance (over 80% on average) and compliance with homework practice using audiotapes, has been good. At the end of the "basic" course there is a relatively unstructured follow-up "drop-in" group for continuing practice of the techniques and maintaining contact with those interested in doing so. Emotional ventilation and supportive discussion is encouraged at both kinds of groups.

This experience has shown the acceptability and apparent usefulness to patients of a simple group training approach: comparison of scores on standard self-report scales show a significant alleviation of anxiety, depression and other psychological symptoms after the basic course compared with 6 weeks earlier, and this is maintained at 3 month follow-up (to be published). We cannot draw any conclusions about effects on survival, but we have the impression that those patients who do well medically seem to be often those who are most involved with their self-help practices. It could be argued that a betterprognosis selects those patients with more interest in self-help practice but this will have to be tested experimentally.

There are several kinds of selection operating: first, the patients who present themselves are volunteers to the programme, and cannot readily be compared with matched non-volunteers, even those with similar disease. Yet we can hardly randomise these volunteers and consign half of them permanently to a control treatment. Furthermore, among those learning self-help methods there is a wide range of intensity with which the work is pursued. Our hypothesis is that those who do most, have, in general, the best chance of affecting the course of their disease.

Both to accommodate these varying needs of patients, and to allow a stratification of patients by "involvement," for research analysis, we are developing a tiered system of groups; reaching basic coping skills at the first level, more in-depth meditation and evolution of personally meaningful imagery at the second, and at the third level, self-study with a psychological journal, exploration of "meaning" of disease and of unconscious resources through guided imagery, and encouragement of extensive daily practice. The therapeutic aim is to provide people with a variety of techniques and levels so that they can take what they want, leaving without regret when they have reached their preferred level.

Difficulties and Limitations of Self-Help

Exaggerated, unsubstantiated claims are often made and this can produce disillusionment in patients and promote a medical backlash. The truth of psychological self-help potential lies somewhere between the poles represented by conservative medicine on the one hand and holistic missionaries on the other.

It must be admitted that self-help is not, and probably never will be, appealing to everyone. For some patients the need to deny the seriousness of their situation, or the secondary gains associated with their illness, preclude a change in attitudes and behaviour while others simply have little wish to live. However, many individuals who have the intrinsic capacity and will to help themselves are unaware of their potential to do so. Western culture is highly materialistic, and generally uncomprehending of mind-body effects; this lowers peoples' expectations and beliefs about what they can do to help themselves and provides an unsympathetic environment for those who try. Because of this climate, self-help is not yet a systematic part of treatment in most conventional hospitals and relatively few patients seek it. Growing awareness will depend on cultural change.

Some clinicians see patients' self-help efforts as an infringement on their "territory." This follows if the patient is seen as a necessarily passive recipient of external care, a view which many patients of course tacitly reinforce at present. Promoting self-help makes better sense against a different philosophical background: that individuals should be encouraged to maximum self-determination in health as in other areas, the role of clinicians being primarily to help rather than to cure.

The issue of the patient's "responsibility" for health is a sensitive one.

Advocating responsibility for personal health is often said to imply blame for ill-health and thus to foster guilt. The other side of the argument, less often expressed, is that responsibility offers freedom for a degree of self-determination. This question must be carefully discussed in professionally-led self-help programmes, which provide an opportunity to moderate the exaggerated claims often found in the popular press.

A related matter is the need to respect patients' defences and wishes for denial of their situation. Seriously weakened patients obviously must not be taxed with learning new techniques and attitudes. The gentle use of relaxation and meditation, presented as coping methods, may nevertheless be useful to most patients, whatever their condition.

Conclusions

There seems to be sufficient justification for introducing programmes teaching self-help as part of the systematic health care of the chronically ill, including many cancer patients. An approach such as that outlined by Achterberg and Lawlis (66) could be followed, presenting these techniques as a way of coping with the disease and aiming primarily to improve quality of life. For selected patients, more "aggressive" intervention would be appropriate in an attempt to counteract the physical disease: these would be people with good ego strength, high motivation and belief in their ability to help themselves, and a willingness to face their situation without undue denial and to make appropriate behaviour changes. The limits to what may be achieved by highly motivated people will have to be established by experiment.

Acknowledgements

I Thank Dr. J.E. Till and Ms. Elizabeth Tocco for reviewing the manuscript and Mrs. Anne Collins for preparing it.

References

1. King, C. (1980). The self-help/self-care concept. Nurse Practitioner, May-June, 34–40.
2. Cassileth, B.R., Lusk, E.J., Strouse, T.B., Bodenheimer, B.J. (1984). Contemporary unorthodox treatments in cancer medicine. Annals of Internal Medicine, 101, 105–112.
3. Arkko, P.J., Arkko, B.L., Kari-Koskinen, O., Taskinen, P.J. (1980). A survey of unproven cancer remedies and their users in an outpatient clinic for cancer therapy in Finland. Social Science and Medicine, 14A, 511–514.

4. Grobstein, C. and Committee. (1982). Diet, Nutrition and Cancer. National Research Council, USA. National Academy Press, Washington, D.C.

5. Doll, R., Peto, R. (1981). The causes of cancer. Journal of the National Cancer Institute, 66, 1191–1308.

6. Moertel, C.G., Fleming, T.R., Rubin, J. et al. (1979). A clinical trial of amygdalin (laetrile) in the treatment of human cancer. New England Journal of Medicine, 306, 201–6.

7. Creagan, E.T., Moertel, C.G., O'Fallon, J.R. et al. (1979). Failure of high dose vitamin C (ascorbic acid) therapy to benefit patients with advanced cancer: a controlled trial. New England Journal of Medicine, 301, 687–90.

8. Moertel, C.G., Fleming, T.R., Creagan, E.T. et al. (1985). High-dose vitamin C versus placebo in the treatment of patients with advanced cancer who have had no prior chemotherapy. New England Journal of Medicine, 312, 137–41.

9. Holland, J.C. (1982). Why patients seek unproven cancer remedies: a psychological perspective. CA-A Cancer Journal for Clinicians, 32, 10–14.

10. Darby, W.J. (1979). Etiology of nutritional fads. Cancer, 43, 2121–4.

11. Janssen, W.F. (1978). The cancer "cures". Analytical Chemistry, 50, 197–202.

12. Peteet, J.R. (1982). A closer look at the concept of support: some applications to the care of patients with cancer. General and Hospital Psychiatry, 4, 19–23.

13. Panagis, D.M. (1979). Supportive therapy: goals and methods. In: Mind and Cancer Prognosis, B.A. Stoll (Ed.), pp. 139–52.

14. Holland, J.C., Rowland, J.H. (1981). Psychiatric, psychosocial and behavioral interventions in the treatment of cancer. In: Perspectives on Behavioral Medicine. S.M. Weiss, (Ed.), Academic Press, New York, pp. 235–260.

15. Freidenbergs, I., Gordon, W., Hibbard, M., Levine, L., Wolf, C., Diller, L. (1981–2). Psychosocial aspects of living with cancer: a review of the literature. International Journal of Psychiatry in Medicine, 11, 303–329.

16. Watson, M. (1983). Psychosocial intervention with cancer patients: a review. Psychological Medicine, 13, 839–46.

17. Spiegel, D., Bloom, J.R., Yalom, I. (1981). Group support for patients with metastatic cancer. Archives of General Psychiatry, 38, 527–533.

18. Yalom, I.D., Greaves, C. (1977). Group therapy with the terminally ill. American Journal of Psychiatry, 134, 396–400.

19. Bloom, J.R., Ross, R.D., Burnell, G. (1978). The effect of social support on patient adjustment after breast surgery. Patient Counselling and Health Education, 1, 50–59.

20. Johnson, J. (1982). The effects of a patient education course on persons with a chronic illness. Cancer Nursing, April, 117–123.

21. Schwartz, M.D. (1977). An information and discussion program for women after a mastectomy. Archives of Surgery, 112, 276–281.

22. Calman, K.C., Welsh, J. (1984). Tak tent: an experiment in self-help for cancer patients. The Practitioner, 228, 585–87.

23. Cobau, C. (1981). The "Life With Cancer" support group at Flower Hospital. Progress in Clinical Biological Research, 57, 177–78.

24. Adams, J. (1979). Mutual-help groups: enhancing the coping ability of oncology clients. Cancer Nursing, April, 95–97.

25. Maisiak, R., Cain, M., Yarbro, C.H., Josof, L. (1981). Evaluation of TOUCH: an oncology self-help group. Oncology Nursing Forum, 8, 20–25.

26. Timothy, F.E. (1980). The Reach to Recovery Program in America and Europe. Cancer, 46, 1059–60.

27. Kelly, O.F. (1975). Make today count. Archives of the Foundation of Thanatology, 5, 461.

28. Iszak, P.C., Engel, J., Medalie, J. (1973). Comprehensive rehabilitation of the patient with cancer.

Five-year experience of a home-care unit. Journal of Chronic Disease, 26, 363–374.

29. Euster, S. (1979). Rehabilitation after mastectomy: the group process. Social Work in Health Care, 4, 251–63.

30. Barish, H. (1971). Self-help groups. Encyclopedia of Social Work, 16, 1163–8.

31. Weisman, A.D., Worden, J.W., Sobel, H.J. (1980). Psychosocial screening and intervention with cancer patients. Research report, Boston. Privately printed.

32. Feinstein, A.D. (1983). Psychological interventions in the treatment of cancer. Clinical Psychology Review, 3, 1–14.

33. Levy, S.M. (1982). Biobehavioral interventions in behavioral medicine. Cancer, 50, 1928–1934.

34. Redd, W.H., Hendler, C.S. (1983). Behavioral medicine in comprehensive cancer treatment. Journal of Psychosocial Oncology, 1, 3–17.

35. Burish, T.G., Carey, M.P. (1984). Conditioned responses to cancer chemotherapy: etiology and treatment. In B.H. Fox and B.H. Newberry (Eds.), Impact of Psychoendocrine Systems in Cancer and Immunity, pp. 147–78. New York: C.J. Hogrefe.

36. Redd, W.H., Rosenberger, P.H., Hendlre, C.S. (1983). Controlling chemotherapy side effects. American Journal of Clinical Hypnosis, 25, 161–72.

37. Gybels, J. Adriaenson, H., Cosyns, P. (1976). Treatment of pain in patients with advanced cancer. European Journal of Cancer, 12, 341–51.

38. Sacerdote, P. (1970). Theory and practice of pain control in malignancy and other protracted or recurring painful illnesses. International Journal of Clinical and Experimental Hypnosis, 18, 160–80.

39. Sacerdote, P. (1978). Teaching self-hypnosis to patients with chronic pain. Journal of Human Stress, 4, 18–21.

40. Orne, M.T. (1974). Pain suppression by hypnosis and related phenomena. In Advances in Neurology. J.J. Bonica (Ed.) New York, Raven Press, pp. 563–579.

41. Barber, J. (1978). Hypnosis as a psychological technique in the management of cancer pain. Cancer Nursing, 1, 361–63.

42. Olness, K. (1981). Imagery (self-hypnosis) as adjunct therapy in childhood cancer. American Journal of Pediatric Hematology/Oncology, 3, 313–21.

43. Jay, S.M., Elliott, C.E. (1983). Psychological intervention for pain in pediatric cancer patients. In Pediatric Oncology, G.B. Humphrey, L.P. Dehner, G.B. Grindley and R.T. Acton. (Eds.) Vol. 3. Boston: Martinus Nijhoff.

44. Spiegel, D., Bloom, J.R. (1983). Group therapy and hypnosis reduce metastatic breast carcinoma pain. Psychosomatic Medicine, 45, 333–39.

45. Turk, D.C., Meichenbaum, D., Genest, M. (1983). Pain and Behavioral Medicine. Guilford Press.

46. Singer, J.E. (1984). Some issues in the study of coping. Cancer, 53, 2303–13.

47. Tarrier, N. (1983). A behavioural approach to the psychological problems of mastectomy. British Journal of Clinical and Social Psychiatry, 2, 41–3.

48. Weisman, A.D., Sobel, H.J. (1979). Coping with cancer through self-instruction: a hypothesis. Journal of Human Stress, March, 3–8.

49. Cameron, E., Pauling, L., Leibovitz, B. (1979). Ascorbic acid and cancer: a review. Cancer Research, 39, 663–81.

50. Cunningham, A.J. (1985). The influence of mind on cancer. Canadian Psychology, 26, 13–29.

51. Benson, H., Epstein, M.D. (1975). The placebo effect. A neglected asset in the care of patients. Journal of American Medical Association, 232, 1225–27.

52. Shapiro, D. (1977). A monologue on biofeedback and psychophysiology. Psychophysiology, 14, 213–27.

53. Bowers, K.S., Kelly, P. (1979). Stress, disease, psychotherapy and hypnosis. Journal of Abnormal Pscyhology, 88, 490–505.

54. Ader, R., Cohen, N. (1975). Behaviorally conditioned immunosuppression. Psychosomatic Medicine, 37, 333–40.

142

55. Simonton, O.C., Mathews-Simonton, S., Creighton, J. (1978). Getting Well Again. J.P. Tarcher, Los Angeles.
56. Achterberg, J., Lawlis, G.F. (1978). Imagery of Cancer. Chicago: Institute for Personality and Ability Testing.
57. Simonton, O.C., Mathews-Simonton, S., Sparks, T.F. (1980). Psychological intervention in the treatment of cancer. Psychosomatics, 21, 226–33.
58. Newton, B.W. (1982–83). The use of hypnosis in the treatment of cancer patients. American Journal of Clinical Hypnosis, 25, 104–13.
59. Meares, A. (1980). What can the cancer patient expect from intensive meditation? Australian Family Physician, 9, 322–25.
60. Meares, A. (1982–83). A form of intensive meditation associated with the regression of cancer. American Journal of Clinical Hypnosis, 25, 114–21.
61. Grossarth-Maticek, R., Schmidt, P., Vetter, H., Arndt, S. (1984). Psychotherapy research in oncology. In: Health Care and Human Behaviour. A. Steptoe and A. Mathews (Eds.), Academic Press, New York, pp. 325–41.
62. Morgenstern, H., Gellert, G.A., Walter, S.D., Ostgeld, A.M., Siegel, B.S. (1984). The impact of a psychosocial support program on survival with breast cancer: the importance of selection bias in program evaluation. Journal of Chronic Disease, 37, 273–82.
63. Shapiro, A. (1982–83). Psychotherapy as adjunct treatment for cancer patients. American Journal of Clinical Hypnosis, 25, 150–55.
64. Weinstock, C. (1977). Notes on "spontaneous" regression of cancer. Journal of American Society of Psychosomatic Dentistry and Medicine 24, 106–110.
65. Mahrer, A.R. (1980). The treatment of cancer through experiential psychotherapy. Psychotherapy: Theory, Research and Practice, 17, 335–42.
66. Achterberg, J., Lawlis, G.F. (1980). Bridges of the Bodymind. Institute for Personality and Ability Testing, Inc., Illinois.

Chapter 15

Caring for Cancer in the Young

MARTIN G. MOTT

Cancer is primarily a disease of the elderly and the proportion of people affected in childhood is very small. Nevertheless, about one person in every 500 will develop malignant disease during the years of childhood and, despite a much improved prognosis, cancer remains the most common disease to kill children. At least one in every 1000 young people entering adult life has been cured of childhood cancer, and the physical and psychological sequelae of the disease and its treatment are therefore matters of concern.

The needs and priorities for somebody whose whole potential lifespan lies before them are clearly quite different from those of an elderly patient in the same situation. The need for parents to be involved in making critical decisions about treatment for children too young to give their own consent, the impact of this responsibility on parents and the effects of the disease and its treatment on siblings are likewise problems that are peculiar to the management of children. The purpose of this chapter is to highlight some aspects of caring for cancer patients which are particularly relevant to the young patient.

Problems at Diagnosis

The immediate reaction of most young parents when told that their child has a form of cancer is to see this as the equivalent of a death sentence. One of the first priorities must therefore be to correct this misunderstanding and to convince them that the majority of children with cancer now become longterm survivors. It is in some sense irrelevant whether the tumour diagnosed in their particular child has a 90% chance of cure, or whether it is one in which less than 10% survive the disease. In either case, their child is faced with a life-threatening illness and it is not possible for anyone to say whether or not that particular child will survive. In both cases, the best chances of survival lie in ensuring that optimal treatment is provided, and it is the promise that this will be the case that is the first step in rehabilitation for the family.

It is a general rule that the ability of people to cope with a new and stressful experience and to deal successfully with it is related to their level of understanding of the problem. It is uncommon nowadays for young parents to have any personal experience of death among their relatives or close friends, and when death becomes a possibility for their own child, their fantasies can become quite paralyzing. It is important to be aware of this if it is to be coped with, because these concerns are rarely brought to the attention of the medical and nursing staff voluntarily

It is advisable to establish a positive and active attitude in the whole family as soon as possible, because when faced with the news that a child in the family has cancer, the natural tendency is to feel helpless, passive prisoners of the situation. The threat of death should therefore be used to concentrate their attention on the value of life, on seeking a cure and of rehabilitation to normal living. Important as such a positive attitude is, it is nevertheless necessary to be realistic and to continue to acknowledge the possibility that death might be the outcome. This becomes increasingly relevant if the disease fails to remit or if relapse occurs, circumstances which make a negative outcome more likely.

Family Orientation

The management of childhood cancer should be organised in a way that enables the child and parents to see that they fulfil a central role in the management team. Unless positive efforts are made to avoid it, the role of parents is all too easy to usurp, and they are left as passive bystanders, angry at their exclusion at a time when all their attention is concentrated on trying to do their best for the child. With care and imagination, a large poroportion of the help that is needed for the child can be channelled through the parents, thus reinforcing their role rather than reducing it.

Of course, it is more difficult and time-consuming to work with a distressed family than simply to do things to or for them. For example, it takes time to educate them in simple day-to-day routines of nursing care that can expand rather than contract their role. The effort is, however, well worth it and such a policy makes a fundamental difference to the well being of the child and the whole family.

A family-oriented approach requires that they be educated about the disease, its treatment, and potential complications. Also about effects that are likely to occur at home and on return to school, and the likely problems that may arise with siblings. Simple pamphlets with a lot of basic information are a helpful starting point, but every family is unique, and their particular methods of coping will depend on their intellectual, emotional and cultural background. There is therefore no substitute for personal instruction by senior members of the medical, nursing and social work staff, with a wealth of past relevant experience to draw from.

Parents

The impact of a life-threatening illness in their child is such that parents are thrown into a tangle of emotions which makes it difficult for them to cope with the many practical problems they are beset with, not least that of maintaining the security and sense of wellbeing of their child. Parents need to be encouraged to talk about their feelings and to be given a simple explanation of the normal grieving process so that they can understand a little about what is happening to them. It can be very comforting to know that those feelings which to them are new, powerful and frightening, are commonplace for people in their situation and do not indicate either an inability to cope or the onset of madness, which is the unspoken fear of many. Among the many emotions which parents experience, feelings of anger and guilt are common and can become destructive. It is important to acknowledge these feelings and to deal with them in a constructive manner.

It is a natural reaction to blanket the threatened child with love, comfort and security. Such attention is something we all find satisfying in the acute phase of an illness, but it can become counterproductive if it persists. In childhood there is a programmed series of steps of developing independence from the safety and security of the family nest, and frustration of this movement is harmful to the wellbeing of the child. This is especially relevant in the adolescent age group.

It is natural to regress a little under the stress of a severe illness, and the nature of the illness itself often enforces increasing dependence on others for one's needs. Parents should be helped to understand that they must discipline their natural inclination to provide all the help and support required by the child. They need instead to foster the independence of the child which is so threatened by his illness.

The child with cancer usually spends a considerable time in hospital, often some distance away from home, and one parent is frequently obliged to take primary responsibility for the sick child, while the other copes with maintaining the rest of the family unit and acting as the breadwinner. An especially close relationship may then begin to develop between the child and parent who are thrust together on their own away from the rest of the family. It is easy in these circumstances for the other partner to feel excluded. Parents should therefore be encouraged to exchange roles as much as possible. They should also be reminded to make sure that they leave enough time for their own relationship, which is inevitably stressed by the separation and by anxiety about their children.

The Child

One of the cardinal features which distinguishes young children as patients from adults is their exquisite sensitivity to non-verbal communication. The general atmosphere surrounding young children treated for cancer is therefore of great importance and every effort must be made to treat them in facilities appropriate to their age and stage of development. Communication with young children is something which comes naturally to some, but is difficult for many. The form in which communication takes place is quite different with someone aged two or twelve or twenty.

Because treatment has so many unpleasant facets, with painful operations and procedures, and drugs or radiation which may cause many unpleasant side effects, it is vital to establish an atmosphere of trust so that the child knows what to expect, and does not spend every waking moment dreading what might be going to happen next. It is widely recognised that in general terms, it is better to share the unpalatable truth than to attempt to cover up the reality of the situation, since children inevitably learn far more of the truth than people think, however expert the attempts to deceive.

Some of the most difficult ethical dilemmas arise in trying to assess how long it is wise or legitimate to persist in attempts to control disease which appears to be progressing, and what level of toxic side effects is tolerable when weighing the pros and cons of a proposed course of action. Here again, the general rule is that even very young children can usually be much more involved in making decisions about their own future than most people give them credit for.

The concerns of children are often quite different from those of adults. One of the most difficult parts of the illness if often having to face returning to school. For children who have lost their hair and are acutely self-conscious about wearing a wig or cap or scarf, this can be a major ordeal. For parents, on the other hand, the biggest concern about a return to school is likely to be the risk of infection. This is frequently overemphasised, because in practice most serious infections in immunosuppressed children with cancer are due to their own endogenous organisms, i.e. staphylococci from their skin and coliforms from their gut: they usually cope as well as anybody else with the common infectious diseases of childhood. The major exceptions to this rule are chickenpox and measles, which can both be fatal, and it is these to which attention should be addressed when encouraging children back to school, and encouraging the school to treat them as far as possible as normal.

Children also fear for their ability to keep up with work because of frequent absences from the classroom, though in practice we find that the teachers in the hospital and school integrate well, and most children more than compensate for their absences in quite a short time. There is a particular bonus in encouraging children to keep up with their schoolwork; it emphasizes to them their prospects for the future.

Death and Dying

Although the results of treatment for childhood cancer have substantially improved in recent decades, an unacceptable proportion of children still die of the disease. When it becomes clear that there is no longer any prospect of cure, it is important that the switch in emphasis to palliative care should not be associated with any sense of abandonment by the treatment team. Children become accustomed to alternating periods at home and in the hospital and are acclimatised to the fact that as new problems arise, so they need to be resolved. They know from experience that periods at home may be required for rest between periods of active treatment.

Home and hospital should not be seen as entirely separate aspects of their lives. When they are hospitalized, it is important to allow them to bring some of their most treasured possessions with them. A strange and often frightening environment can thereby be made more familiar and reassuring. Similarly, those parts of the hospital environment which are important to them for comfort and security may need to be transported with them into the home. The most important aspects of their sense of security are often those people they have grown to know and trust, and this can be the most difficult problem to resolve if they live a considerable distance from the hospital. Most families prefer to nurse a dying child at home provided they can feel confident that this is the best place for the child. This means ensuring that expert advice on the terminal care of children is available to them 24 hours a day from the hospital staff, working in close collaboration with the primary care team.

A process of anticipatory mourning is natural, but can sometimes get in the way of the provision of the loving care and attention which the child needs during this time. The re-investment of parental time and energy away from the child may need to be slowed and controlled, or it may become a focus of contention among the surviving members of the family at a later date. Sensitive and knowledgeable counselling is crucial at this stage.

Many parents are left with agonising doubts and uncertainties about often minor and unimportant details concerning their child's death. Most of these can be resolved by getting together to discuss the results of an autopsy examination a few weeks after the event. The worst time to approach parents about an autopsy is immediately after the death of their child; this subject should have been skilfully introduced into the conversation some considerable time beforehand, so that they will have had time to weigh up the possible advantages to themselves and to others in agreeing to an autopsy, and to adjust to the idea that it will not involve further suffering for the child. Some parents feel unable to face a return visit to the hospital in the immediate weeks after their child has died and it may be necessary to arrange an alternative venue to meet.

Many parents face major problems when they find that even close family and friends are embarrassed to talk about the child who has died. They often draw great strength and consolation at this time from the therapeutic community of professionals and other parents whom they have come to regard as an extended family during the treatment period. The provision of aftercare by alternative professionals who did not know their child and had no part in their management, seems a poor substitute but regretfully, it is often all that is available to them.

Chapter 16

Caring for the Family

KERRY BLUGLASS

In examining the potential needs of the relatives of the patient with cancer, we must aim for a flexible approach to that group of people we might call the family. We must consider not only the "conventional family" (1), but also any other individuals who are "key persons" (2) in the life of that patient. When a group of individuals is clustered together in what we call a family, we can no more expect any one particular response to stress than we could expect a standard or stereotyped response from one individual. Nevertheless, there are certain patterns which recur, both in the individual and in groups of people, which we can learn to recognise and which will enable us to help our patients and their relatives.

We need to understand the usual reaction of most healthy adults to threat, loss and change (3, 4, 5), in order to appreciate how people generally behave in the anticipation of these events. We also need some understanding of the different reactions of children in the family and how these are coloured by the developmental age of the child. Thus, we must free ourselves from preconceptions based upon adult behaviour before we can begin to anticipate the whole family's response under stress.

Characteristics of the Family

In considering the reactions of any particular family, it is helpful to look at the structure and function of the family in general. Although we retain an image of what the sociologists would call a conventional family (1), changes have occurred in kinship and marriage patterns, geographical mobility, divorce legislation, employment and acceptance of single parenthood of either sex. The realities of social changes have certain implications for our view of the typical family.

In the USA, the departure from established family patterns because of distance, separation or divorce is becoming familiar. In Europe on the other hand (particularly in non-industrialised parts), family and kinship patterns are often much more traditional. In Catholic countries, divorce or family break-up is somewhat less common, and acceptance of the elderly or sick parent as the natural responsibility of the individual and community is also more traditional.

There are undeniable advantages in this way of life, but some hidden problems too. For example, in some European countries there is a resignation to fate which we may find hard to grasp, and community and social attitudes to death and bereavement are perhaps more like those of Britain of the 19th century. Although the support of the Church and organised religious framework are helpful for mourning, there is less community understanding of the social role of widow and widower, and identification of those bereaved people with special needs. Improving public expectation and professional education by writing, teaching, conferences and professional interchange (6) will be as important as the slower process of social change.

We should remind ouselves that a "key person" (2) may be much more important than a distant but biologically nearer relative. By reason of his or her psychological relationship to the patient, he or she may be the most "at risk" in the event of the death of the patient: as for example, in a homosexual relationship which may be equal in closeness and duration to that of many marriages. If unrecognised for fear of social disapproval, the surviving partner may be deprived of the accepted social support accorded to a spouse.

Consideration of the functions of the family go beyond assessments as to whether the family is reasonably cohesive and close, or able to unite in adversity whatever the previous differences of opinion. It should look at the functional position of each family member (7), meaning the role which the person occupies in that family. Family members may take up (or be assigned) roles such as "the scapegoat," the "value setter" or "the head of the clan." The illness or death of this person will leave a gap, not only of the physical presence, but of the place fulfilled by this person and a corresponding gap in the dynamic balance of the family. The needs of a family with a young child with cancer are considered in the previous chapter, but young children play an important part in the dynamic balance of a family and their deaths will alter this balance.

Aims of Family Support

We not only have to decide who needs support, but also what the support is to involve. We must be certain that it is positive, constructive and affirming of the family or individual's strengths, rather than encouraging weakness and dependency which in future could lead to loss of coping skills. When a relative has been perfectly able to do small domestic or personal tasks for the patient at home, it is a diminution of his or her abilities if professionals take over all of these roles in hospital. This is an example of the valuable potential of preventive work for the survivor.

Relatives who continue to wash, feed, dress the patient in hospital as they did at home are likely to preserve their self-esteem better, and face eventual loss and bereavement with a better outcome, less guilt and self reproach. They should be allowed (wherever possible clinically) to do so even if this may call for some rethinking, modification and flexibility of our ward practices. It is almost always possible, if we are prepared to change and to be creative in our care for patients to allow both patient and relative much greater autonomy than we imagine. The aim should be to give back to the patient and relative the sense of "mastery" which they would have at home.

It is salutary sometimes to stop and ask our patients' families about the practical aspects of visiting the ward daily, often from a great distance. It is often assumed that the Social Worker will deal with matters such as financial hardship, transport and other practical matters, but the "wear and tear" factor should never be underestimated. Quite apart from the physical "drain," the death of a patient after a long period of exhausting visiting or vigil may produce understandable feelings of relief, which may be misunderstood by staff as indifference or lack of concern. This "paradoxical" relief may worsen the inevitable feelings of guilt in bereavement, leading to development of later difficulties. Even the strains involved in keeping other interested family members abreast of clinical changes in the patient's condition can be overwhelming, and can add to the burden of the need for frequent visiting.

The need for the relatives to balance regular visits to a patient in hospital with the competing demands of well family members and the commitments of employment are all sources of additional strain on the family. They may lead to guilt and resentment directed at the patient but hard to express. For this reason, irritation may be voiced uncharacteristically either at work, with other family members or towards members of the team caring for the patient. Anger may also surface towards the staff who "break bad news" (8).

Stress may result from blood relationship to the patient. Relatives may have fears concerning heredity (breast cancer, for example) which need to be discussed openly. An identical twin of a woman with terminal cervical cancer has fears for her own health, but also needs support in confirming her own identity after her twin's death.

In some families the "sick role" of the patient becomes a mutually suitable way of life. For example, it may suit an overprotective parent to have an ailing partner or child, and this can make a return to health either in remission or in the long term, an uncomfortable process. Such a situation can explain apparently paradoxical behaviour, such as the family member who refuses to accept a good or improving prognosis, or a marital break-down which fails to occur during the stressful period of illness but occurs once the prognosis improves.

There are special phases of the illness which may cause difficulties for the family, and one obvious example is the unexpected remission. It is not uncommon to see a terminal situation in which hope of a longer life has been abandoned, further efforts in active treatment relinquished, "acceptance" accomplished, and many or all of the psychological tasks involved in anticipating loss worked through. Death is recognised to be not far off – and yet the patient continues to live on, and sometimes (as a consequence of illness or treatment) is also radically changed in appearance or behaviour.

This can be an intolerable source of distress to the patient and relatives, and since it will often be hard to express for reasons of loyalty, staff members should be alert to indications of its existence. A practical way to help is to ask the family to show past photographs and this will allow them to talk about changes in appearance.

In any phase of the illness (but especially when it is assumed that active treatment is no longer appropriate) great psychological distress may arise from the need to reconcile family members or carry out important legal or administrative affairs. In these circumstances, the family and the team of clinicians may need to review the previous plan of therapeutic action or inaction, in order to "buy time," for example to allow for the visit of a distant relative or for old quarrels to be settled. To do so can make great improvements in bereavement outcome since ambivalent or stormy relationships are known to be risk factors in mourning (9, 10).

Families may collude to keep feelings at a distance or suppress them, and may keep individual members from expressing them. After a death there are often many emotions which must be expressed, including the need to cry and to recognise that anger may be an appropriate emotion in certain circumstances. To "bottle it up" can be as destructive as the need in other circumstances to leave it behind.

Recent techniques developed to help express emotion include a technique known as "Guided Mourning" (11), one that may be very useful when appropriate responses in bereavement are hindered or blocked by certain psychological barriers. It is however not suitable for use in other than skilled and experienced hands.

Techniques of Intervention

Helping the family does not necessarily mean doing things for them, but may involve the family in learning to do things for itself. Many of the techniques in Family Therapy Practice (12) are exercised in highly specialised form by experienced workers, but the principles can be learned and applied in the help which can be given to a family group. Thus, one may appreciate the strengths and the risks inherent in some family situations by constructing a Genogram (a diagrammatic representation of family members past and present, and their relationships to one another). One can easily see how the removal of a member by illness or death will alter the balance of the family.

Family re-grouping will occur after a death, and often during the actual illness of a family member. If this occurs inappropriately (for example, a daughter being cast in the role of "mother" or a son expected to be "the man" where intellectually, emotionally or developmentally this is inappropriate), the balance may be shifted. "Equilibrium" of sorts may be regained by socially inappropriate behaviour, physical or emotional illness or disability.

Should support of patients and their families be on an individual or on a group basis? While some prefer one to the other, the final determinant must be the method which is likely to be most beneficial to the family. Johnson (13) has described a method of evaluating "consumer satisfaction" in a group programme for cancer patients and family members.

Group methods of support in bereavement have grown out of considerations of cost-effectiveness, but in suitable situations can provide shared experience and mutual support. When appropriately led, they go beyond that which can be provided by the professional, but the term "appropriately led" requires explanation. Parkes (14) stresses that an objective professional leader is necessary not only to bring the skills of group leadership to bear, but also to identify destructive processes such as anger, bitterness, or over-involvement which can impede the progress of other members of the group and hinder their recovery. A professional leader will also identify the need for further specialised referral.

Other techniques include conventional psychiatric or psychological techniques, such as crisis intervention. Berger (15) has described an open "drop-in" group for patients and families aimed at promoting adaptive responses. Such groups can be easily generalised, into good psychosocial support systems as adjuncts to oncology units.

Behavioural modification techniques for specific problems are also used (16). As with other techniques, a behavioural approach (usually accessible to the team through a clinical psychologist) is applicable to problems presenting in patient or family at any stage of the illness. The principle and techniques can be learned and applied by all members of the team. An interesting research tool with practical implications has recently been described by Goldberg (17), and involves a manual for teaching and evaluating counselling techniques suitable for brief psychotherapy with patients' spouses.

Conclusion

We need to strengthen ways of coping with stress in the family of the cancer patient, and support both patients and relatives in a spirit of optimism so that they are able to keep control of their affairs. Support must be tailored to the individual need, and very often that means to support the strengths already present, not take over the direction of people's lives.

Future activity in the field of family support must include more reports of good practice, and evaluation of the increasing range of different methods of support. It seems likely that the consumer – patients and families – will speak with an increasingly clear voice and we must ensure that this is heard.

References

1. Oakley, A. (1982), Conventional families. In: Families in Britain (Eds. R.N. Rapoport, M.P. Fogarty). Routledge & Kegan Paul. London.
2. Parkes, C.M. (1984). Psychological Aspects. In: The Management of Terminal Malignant Disease (Ed. C.M. Saunders). Edward Arnold, London
3. Marris, P. (1974) Loss and Change. Routledge and Kegan Paul, London
4. Parkes, C.M., Weiss, R.S. (1983). Recovery from Bereavement. Basic Books, New York.
5. Parkes, C.M. (1972). Bereavement. Penguin, Harmondsworth.
6. World Health Organisation (1984). Guidelines for the Relief of Cancer pain, World Health Organisation, Geneva.
7. Worden, J.W. (1983). Grief and Family Systems. In Grief Counselling and Grief Therapy, Tavistock, London.
8. Buckman, R. (1984). Breaking bad news. Why is it so difficult? British Medical Journal 288, 1592-9.
9. Stedeford, A. (1984). Bereavement: complicated grief. In Facing Death – Patients, Families and Professionals, Heinemann Medical, London.
10. Primary Health Care for Cancer Patients (1983). In Royal College of Psychiatrists Evidence to the DHSS working group on cancer.
11. Mawson, D., Marks, I.M., Ramm, L., and Stern (1981). Guided mourning for morbid grief. British Journal of Psychiatry, 138, 185-93.
12. Minuchin, S. (1974). Families and family therapy. Tavistock, London.
13. Johnson, E.M., Stark, D.E. (1980). A group program for cancer patients and their family members in an acute care teaching hospital. Social Work and Health Care, 5, 335-49.
14. Parkes, C.M. (1980). Bereavement counselling does it work? British Medical Journal, 281, 3-6.
15. Berger, J.M. (1984). Crisis intervention: A drop-in support group for cancer patients and their families. Social Work and Health Care, 10, 81-92.
16. Heinrich, R.L., Schag, C.C. (1984). A behavioural medicine approach to coping with cancer: a case report. Cancer Nursing, 1, 243-7.
17. Goldberg, R.J., Wool, M., Tull, R., Boor, M. (1984). Teaching brief psychotherapy for spouses of cancer patients: use of a codable supervision format. Psychotherapy and Psychosomatics, 41, 12-19.

Chapter 17

Caring for the Terminal Patient

MARGARET W. LINN AND BERNARD S. LINN

People face death in many different ways. Counselling may help some while others prefer to meet death in their own private way; helping a person face death starts with this recognition of individual style. Thus, our own values concerning what needs to be done should not be imposed and the person's own wishes are to be respected above all else.

Role of the Physician

The physician plays a significant role for dying patients, but personal or organizational bariers may impede this aspect of care (1). Such barriers may include limited knowledge, skill or motivation, apart from lack of time or staff support. The majority of physicians in practice today have unfortunately received little or no education in the art of meeting the needs of the dying and their families (2). In general, they are concerned more with bodily function than with the whole person (3) and they are not educated to ease the distress of dying (4). Some physicians even perceive death of a patient as a personal failure and professional defeat (5).

Traditionally, it used to be the family doctor who helped the patient make the transition between life and death, while offering support and comfort to the patient's family as well. But the technological advances in medicine, including the development of hospitals and nursing homes (as well as changes in the family structure over the past quarter century) have resulted in patients sometimes being isolated from others in their last few weeks of life. Patients are now more likely to die in hospitals than at home, and the practice of medicine in our specialized hospitals tends to focus more on curing than on caring.

Recently, the medical profession has shown renewed interest in quality of life as an issue in treatment, instead of aiming at extending life at all costs. This shift is reflected in such measures as the "living will" (6), in which patients can ensure that no heroic procedures will be taken to prolong their lives. Interest in working with the dying is also evidenced by the growing number of seminars which are intended to help hospital personnel recognize their own fears of death and the needs of the dying patient.

Lack of education in dealing with death and dying is evident in many medical schools, and for many students, the first exposure to death is an impersonal one that takes place in the anatomy laboratory. Olin (7) reported that death was seen by medical students as a failure instead of being valued as a dignified event. Attitudes to death may even influence the choice of career and Feifel (8) postulates that some physicians chose a career in medicine because they had a need to master high levels of fear about death by gaining power to cure, control disease, and save lives. He found practising physicians to be more fearful of death than medical students, and medical students more fearful than nonmedical students. While Feifel suggested that continued experience in medicine did not lessen the fear of death but rather enhanced it, Lester and his co-workers (9) found fear of death and dying to decrease with increased academic experiences both for nursing students and faculty members.

Self-selection of careers on the basis of attitudes to death, as well as other personality characteristics, is suggested also by Livingston and Zimet (10). They reasoned that medical students with high feelings of authoritarianism would have few unconscious fears in specialties where death was relatively common, for example in surgery. Students low in authoritarianism, however, would be more uncomfortable by their death anxiety and as a result would choose specialties such as psychiatry, where death was a less common event. These hypotheses were confirmed by their study.

Fear of Death and Dying

Fear of death, or death anxiety, is present in all people to varying degrees, and there is nothing inherently abnormal about it. Attitudes to death should be distinguished from attitudes to dying, which has been described as an event that takes place over a period of time (11). Dying may be painful, emotionally and physically, and is therefore, realistically portrayed as a fearful experience while death is characterized by absence of experience.

We have examined the impact of clinical experience on attitudes of junior medical students to see how their clinical experiences affected attitudes to death and dying (12). They did not change significantly in attitudes toward the dying patient but became more negative about dealing with the dying patient's family.

Students who scored high on personality rigidity had more negative attitudes and changed less during the clerkship. Students who selected more clinically-oriented careers had more positive attitudes than did students who were undecided about careers or were interested more in research, teaching, or nonclinical medical specialties. The results suggest the need for instruction in that field during the clinical years when students are experiencing their first interactions with dying patients and their families.

Dying can be regarded as the ultimate and final stress that an individual has to face. It is one for which some people attempt to prepare during life, while for others it is something they try to avoid on a conscious level. But a diagnosis of cancer unsettles both the emotionally-prepared as well as the unprepared. Patients and their families may face the following problems in the presence of disseminated cancer: (a) high probability of progressive disability; (b) progressive increase in symptom complexity with the sequential involvement of several body systems; (c) progressively more refractory pain; (d) more limited therapeutic resources with only transient efficacy; (e) probability of death after a limited time; (f) discontinuity in medical care which adds substantially to the burdens of the patient, family and physician (13).

If it is not possible to cure the patient and return him to normal life, the goal is to control the disease for as long as possible, and if all else fails, to make the dying patient comfortable and his death painless. A major problem is that modern medical care is geared mainly to acute high intensity care with some attention to low intensity long-term care, but little to the high intensity, long-term type of care that may be needed for cancer patients. The frustration of cancer-afflicted families, seemingly abandoned by institutions they had trusted, is great. The families have no way of knowing that the unresponsiveness they encounter is due more to limited facilities than to lack of concern – limitation in hospital stay, limited help for outpatient costs, limited ability to make home care feasible.

Reactions to Dying

It is a common observation that among cancer patients with approximately identical lesions, degree of dissemination and treatment, some seem to survive far longer than others. Weisman and Worden (14) have shown that longer-than-expected survival tended to occur in patients who had good relationships with others; accepted the reality of their illness, but did not seem to believe that death was inevitable; were seldom depressed; and refused to let others pull away from them. On the other hand, those with shorter survivals had poor social relationships (beginning with early separations from their family and continuing throughout life) were very much more depressed and sometimes suicidal, and often wanted to die.

What makes a good death as opposed to one filled with anguish, depression, despair, and confusion? Within the limits of disability, a patient should function as effectively as possible, should recognize and resolve residual conflict, and satisfy whatever remaining wishes are consistent with his self-concept. Lacking this, the alternative is aimlessness. People without hope see no end to their suffering. Hope involves confidence in the "desirability" of survival, and arises from having a good self-concept and a belief in one's ability to exert some control on the surrounding world.

The common negative emotional responses aroused by cancer are anxiety (fear, dread), anger (frustration, rage), and depression (guilt, despair). Denial of the event, withdrawal, rejection of others, bargaining, and at times true acceptance may be seen. Kubler-Ross (15) discussed five phases that the patient may go through: "Not me (denial); "Why me?" (anger); "Yes, me but ..." (bargaining for time); "Yes, me" (depression), and hopefully, near the end, acceptance of the inevitable. But there is immense variation among patients; some enter and leave one phase a number of times or may never experience more than one or two phases or may skip phases.

Cramond (16) believes that the dying patient does not fear death as much as the process of dying, and suggests that depression, anger, and regression are all major points to consider in the management of the dying patient. Weisman (17) suggests there are levels of dying and denying, and believe that patients can be helped at each stage by psychosocial support.

Kastenbaum and Aisenburg (18) suggest that the dying patient wants to talk, keep communication open, and have a part in the management of his death, while the taboos of death may isolate fatally ill patients so that they are treated as if they are already dead. When counsellors respond to the needs of the terminally ill, there is a beneficial influence on self-esteem, alienation, and depression. This suggests that if physicians and hospital staff members were trained to perceive and meet the needs of the terminally ill, the quality of life and caring during the final days of the patients might be improved immeasurably.

Helping the Dying

Few controlled studies have examined the effectiveness of working with the dying. Over a three-year period, we have evaluated its efectiveness in dying cancer patients by assessing changes in quality of life, physical functioning, and survival (19). One hundred twenty men with end-stage cancer were randomly assigned to experimental or control groups; the 62 experimental group patients were seen regularly by a counsellor. Patients were assessed before random assignment and again at one, three, six, nine, and 12 months, with regard to quality of life and functional status. Counseled patients improved significantly more than the control group with regard to quality of life within three months, but functional status and survival did not differ between groups.

Since it was found possible to influence quality of life positively through counseling, it raised the question of whether training staff members in the principles employed in counselling might change their attitudes and influence quality of life in dying patients. Community nursing homes were selected as a site for training because many patients go to these homes to die, and staff in the homes are less well trained than staff in hospitals. The aim of the study was to test the effects of a training program both on the nursing home personnel and on the patients assigned to their care.

Ten community nursing homes were assigned randomly to training or control conditions. With regard to staff members, training was found to have increased their knowledge and changed their attitudes positively, but to have also increased their anxiety about their own death (20). With regard to patients, 306 terminally ill patients admitted to 10 homes were assessed at the time of admission and again at one and three months later. Patients in the "trained" homes had less depression and greater satisfaction with care at one and three months, compared with patients in the control homes (21). The study indicates that some impact on patient care can be achieved when staff in nursing homes are trained to work with dying patients.

Specific measures to help the dying must be tailored to meet each patient's need. The physician must often decide whether or not to tell the patient about suspected impending death. Even when the dying person suspects that death might occur shortly, the pronouncement itself is unsettling. There is no hard and fast rule saying that all patients should be told; some want to know, others do not. The clue generally comes from the patient. Does the patient ask about what is expected? Does the patient persist in questioning the physician about what is going to happen? If so, the patient probably wants to know.

At the same time, it should be recognized that the physician is not omniscient. Even though there may be little doubt that a condition is fatal, it is difficult – if not impossible – to predict how long a person will live. Therefore, some uncertainty about the time of death and some hope for life can be maintained, even in the face of dying. But just because a patient does not ask about impending death does not mean that he or she is unaware of what is happening.

Listening with empathy may be all that is required. For the busy physician, no more than this may realistically be offered but a counsellor may be able to go further. It does not require firsthand knowledge of an experience in order to share another person's feelings. One may never have made a trip around the world, but it would not be difficult to celebrate the anticipation of such a venture with another person. In a similar way, one can empathize with sorrow, depression, fear, expectation, or any other human emotion expressed by the dying. It is the human contact and the relationship that matters most, and it is wrong to close off all avenues for listening or discussing feelings by telling patients that they should not feel as they do, or to try and reassure them that they are not dying.

When dying takes place over a period of time, there is often a tendency to isolate the person as if already dead. In a hospital, nurses and attendants may answer calls from the patient more slowly and less time is spent with the patient. Physicians and nurses begin to talk in the presence of the patient as if he or she were just a case, and not a person who can hear or understand. Even families may visit less often, becoming more involved in putting their life together, as if the dying relative were already gone. Although the family must do this eventually, the tendency to initiate the process before the person dies – because it excludes the dying – may be seen by the patient as abandonment.

Encouraging the person to reminisce in what Butler (22) has called the "life review" is a particularly helpful process for the elderly. It enables the person to look back over his or her life and develop a sense of meaning. Reviewing the past provides a basis for increased self-esteem and life satisfaction and encouraging the life review during the dying process can thus improve the overall quality of remaining survival.

Helping the dying plan for what they want to accomplish in the time they have left may encourage activities that are especially meaningful for them. Many elderly have not planned for their last days and may wish to complete unfinished business, to resolve some interpersonal family problems, to seek religious guidance, to make their will, or to plan for the disposition of their body after death. Meaningful activities should be encouraged for as long as possible. The dying should have a feeling that they have a part in decisions and some control over their immediate environment. They can share in decisions about their medical treatment. They may be of help to their family in planning finances, in plans for education of children or grandchildren, or in other personal matters. Even though control over the long-range future is lost because of the illness, control over short-range circumstances can be encouraged.

If the patient wants to talk with the family about dying, this also should be encouraged. Families often need to know how they can be of help. Families may need to talk with a counsellor separately about the person's illness or may need help in understanding the normal reactions to dying. It is sometimes helpful to see the dying person and family together and the aim is to keep communication open in the family. Counsellors frequently continue to see the family after the patient's death and may help with emotional support during the process of grieving and readjustment. Unresolved grief in relatives may lead to illness, and possibly accelerate the death of a spouse.

Lastly, communicating without words is always possible. A touch and a warm smile from the physician can mean a lot to the patient. Sometimes a counsellor may simply sit with the patient without talking. Talk may not be necessary – the comfort of having someone who cares nearby cannot be overestimated. Touching the person lightly on the arm or shoulder can convey one's feelings and reassure the person that he or she is touchable and that communication and understanding exist even at this most basic level.

References

1. Harris, R., Hartner, R., Linn, M.W., Linn, B.S. (1979). The importance of the doctor to the dying patient. Southern Medical Journal 72, 1319–1323.

2. Dickinson, G.E. (1981). Death education in U.S. medical schools: 1975–1980. Journal of Medical Education 56, 111–114.

3. Neale, R.E. (1973). The art of dying. Harper and Row, New York.

4. Hackett, T.P. (1976). Psychological assistance for the dying patient and his family. Annual Review of Medicine 5, 371–378.

5. Barton, D. (1972). The need for including instruction on death and dying in the medical curriculum. Journal of Medical Education 47, 169–175.

6. "Living will:" Instruction for my care in the event of terminal illness. American Protestant Hospital Association, Chicago.

7. Olin, H.S. (1982). A proposed model to teach medical students the care of the dying patient. Journal of Medical Education 47, 564–567.

8. Feifel, H. (1976). Toward death: a psychological perspective. Death: Current Perspectives. (Ed. E.S. Shneidman). Mayfield Publishing Co, Palo Alto, California.

9. Lester, D., Getty, L., Kneisl, C.R. (1974). Attitudes of nursing students and nursing faculty toward death. Nursing Research 23, 50–53.

10. Livingston, P.B., Zimet, C.N. (1965). Death anxiety, authoritarianism and choice of specialty in medical students. Journal of Nervous and Mental Disease 140: 222–230.

11. Walton, D. *1976). On the rationality of fear of death. Omega 7, 1–9.

12. Linn, B.S., Moravec, J., Zeppa, R. (1982). The impact of clinical experience on junior medical students' attitudes about death and dying. Journal of Medical Education 57, 684–691.

13. Brennan, M.J. (1970). The cancer gestalt. Geriatrics 25, 96–101.

14. Weisman, A.D., Worden, J.S. (1975). Psychosocial analysis of cancer deaths. Omega 6, 61–75.

15. Kubler-Ross, E. (1969). On Death and Dying. MacMillan Co. New York.

16. Cramond, W.A. (1970). Psychotherapy of the dying patient. British Medical Journal 3, 389–393.

17. Weisman, A.D. (1970). On Dying and Denying. Behavioral Publications, New York.

18. Kastenbaum, R. Aisenburg, R. (1972). The Psychology of Death. Springer, New York.

19. Linn, M.W., Linn, B.S., Harris, R. (1982). Effects of counseling for late stage cancer patients. Cancer 49, 1084–1055.

20. Linn, M.W., Linn, B.W., Stein, S. (1983). Impact on nursing home staff of training about death and dying. Journal of the American Medical Association 250, 2332–2335.

21. Linn, M.W., B.S., Stein, S. (1985). Impact on the patients of training nursing home staff about death and dying (Part II). Journal of the American Medical Association (in review).

22. Butler, R.N. (1964). The life review – an interpretation of reminiscence in the aged. In New Thought on Old Age. Springer, New York.

PART THREE

PERSONAL VIEWPOINTS

Chapter 18

Communicating with the Patient

ROBERT BUCKMAN

In general, the medical profession is not good at communicating with seriously ill patients and their relatives. I would suggest that this is not because we are unsympathetic but because we are not trained for it, and this chapter aims to identify the major difficulties and to suggest ways in which they might be overcome. Many of the problems are common to doctors, nurses and others involved in the care of ill and dying patients, but I shall put most emphasis on the doctor's role, because breaking bad news is usually regarded as a doctor's job and if he does it badly, it makes the situation difficult for everyone else.

Although a lot has been written about the patient's reactions when confronting bad news or the prospect of death, very little has been written (other than in specialist journals) about the doctor's feelings as he attempts to break bad news. Some of the difficulties arise because we are trained to deal systematically with physical illness in a way that makes it difficult for us to know how to behave when different services are required by our patients.

First, some definition of bad news is required. I propose a pragmatic definition of bad news as any news which materially alters a patient's view of his or her future. Naturally, how bad the news seems will depend to some extent on the patient's expectations at the time, or on how ill they feel; also on whether or not they already know or suspect their diagnosis or current state. From this point of view, it may be easier to break bad news when a patient has already made some adjustment to the illness (for example, at the time of first recurrence some years after primary treatment) than it is when the patient has no suspicion that anything is seriously wrong (at the time of diagnosis). For this reason I shall suggest at the end of this chapter that we should not begin discussing bad news until we have some idea of what the patient already knows of the illness, how serious he thinks it is and whether or not he would actually like to have the information given and discussed.

Several studies have shown that at least half of all patients with cancer would like to know the diagnosis, implying that we should be prepared to overcome our own fears and anxieties sufficiently to have a discussion, even if it is not required on every occasion. Thus, in analysing why doctors often fail at this kind of communication. I am not advocating full and detailed discussion with every patient regardless of their wishes, but only that we should have the ability to do it and should offer the opportunity for it to every one of our patients.

I shall consider the obstacles that make discussions difficult under two headings: first, the fears and anxieties that we have that make it awkward for us to begin a conversation; second, the factors that tend to push us into feeling responsible for the bad news itself. The latter makes conversation even more difficult once it has started.

Personal Fears that Doctors May Have

Fears of talking about unpleasant subjects are common to everyone and can perhaps be labelled 'personal' fears. On the other hand, I believe that while we are being trained to deal with medical crises we inadvertently acquire other fears which make it difficult for us to help our patients when our therapeutic skills have nothing to offer. I shall consider these two groups of anxieties separately, although they obviously operate together. First, the personal fears.

Fear of Causing Pain and Taking Away Hope

Breaking bad news causes pain and most people are naturally reluctant to inflict pain on others. This common feeling is of course amplified by medical training during which we are taught to alleviate pain whenever possible, and to use as much analgesia or anaesthesia as required whenever it is necessary to inflict pain. Unfortunately, there is no simple effective analgesic for the pain caused by bad news, so that many doctors avoid the situation altogether.

Loss of hope is one specific example of the pain caused by bad news, and I emphasise it because it can become an excuse for not talking to patients about their illnesses.

The rationale may go something like this 'it is cruel to take away hope, but I can't talk truthfully about the illness without taking away hope, and I don't want to tell lies, so therefore I can't talk to the patient at all.' Experienced workers in this field know that it is possible for patients to talk about their fears and anxieties, and that doing this does not necessarily extinguish hope. Studies have shown that there are more patients who suffer from fear and a sense of isolation because they are unable to discuss their illness with someone, than there are patients who regret such a discussion subsequently.

With a modicum of skill and some understanding of patients' needs, a discussion can help a patient face and adapt to bad news, and the doctor can be seen as the ally of the patient rather than as the person inflicting the pain of taking away hope. I believe that many of us are tempted to use the fear of taking away hope as an excuse for not talking to the patient about the problems uppermost in his mind. I would suggest that although we may reassure ourselves that we are being kind to the patient by doing this, this may not be the case.

Fear of Being Blamed

The worst fear for most doctors – particularly junior doctors – is that the patient will blame them personally for the bad news that they bring. The phenomenon of identifying the bad news with the bearer of it is not new, nor is it unique to doctors (after all, the execution of bad news messengers was quite common in ancient times). I think that this may be a basic trait of human behaviour – coping with bad news in the abstract is very difficult, and it is easier to deal with it when it has a human shape. For example, one gets angry with a traffic warden when the real anger is directed at the parking ticket. It is easier to transfer blame for the bad news onto the bearer if he is readily identifiable – the more conspicuous the uniform and the official authority by which the news arrives, the more readily the blame can be transferred.

Since we all know that transferring blame is a common and socially acceptable way of behaving, doctors must expect and fear this kind of reaction from our patients when it's our turn to wear the badge of authority and hand out the bad news. Worse still, the closer we get to our patients the easier we make it for them to blame us. We are usually easily identifiable, often in uniform, and we hand out important information to our patients. It's easy to see how patients come to regard doctors as the source of *everything* that happens to them. The more authority we have, the more we select ourselves as targets.

Not every patient responds to bad news by blaming the doctor, but it is common and well enough known for many doctors to hesitate before they start the conversation, and possibly to avoid the conversation altogether. Even doctors with many years of experience may find themselves relieved when a patient says "actually I knew it was cancer anyway" and the moment passes without blame. This sense of blame may be very off-putting to doctors and nurses early in their training, and it requires a great deal of schooling to remind ouselves that the patient's disease is not our fault, and therefore that being blamed is a reaction to be taken into account but not to be taken personally.

Fear of Illness and Death

Personal attitudes to death are dealt with in the previouschapter but here two important factors need to be mentioned. One is the social taboo of talking about death, which is a fairly recent and much discussed phenomenon. The other concerns the denial of illness and death by doctors. Some psychologists suggest that the reason for taking up a medical career is the feeling of invulnerability that comes from working among the sick while being healthy. Whether this is a major or a minor motive, it is certainly much easier to defend the illusion of invulnerability by keeping at a distance from the patient.

Fears Acquired during Medical Training

The fears that we acquire during medical training are almost more important than those we already possess as human beings. First, we are very conscious of our training – it's expensive and prolonged and the habits we pick up during our training are often so powerful that we tend to be very resistant to abandoning them. Hence, the fears we acquire along with the useful and appropriate skills are highly reinforced. These fears can be changed and, if we are aware of them, we can alter the medical school curriculum.

Fear of Facing Therapeutic Failure

Most of the medical school curriculum is dedicated to the diagnosis and correction of organic conditions, and this is appropriate. The problem is that so much time is spent on these aspects of training that medical students do not realise that a lot of their time will be spent dealng with situations where their knowledge of therapeutics has little to offer. A person who is unprepared for therapeutic failure will find it unpleasant, and will avoid that patient in favour of one for whom therapeutic skill may be of value.

While we all want to treat treatable conditions, we need to be taught early in our careers how to help patients for whom conventional therapeutics have little to offer. That way, we may realise that facing therapeutic failure is another part of the job of being a doctor – and one in which skill can be acquired and is much appreciated by the patient.

Fear of the Unknown and Untaught

As we get skilful at doing the things we have been taught, we come to feel more and more awkward in situations that we have not been trained for, and this includes talking to dying patients. Only in recent years have medical schools started anytraining in communication skills, so that most doctors will not have been given any guidelines in this difficult area. This means that when trying to talk to patients in this situation they miss the comfort and security of following a course of action that they've been taught.

This fear and avoidance of things we haven't been trained for means that any areas that are out of bounds while we are being trained, stay out of bounds once we are trained. It is as if a subject that is not on the curriculum is not a 'proper' subject for real doctors. This feeling of venturing out beyond the pale of standard medical practice when we are discussing bad news with a patient surely adds to the insecurity and anxiety of an already awkward task.

Fear of Unleashing a Reaction

There is also the problem of what may happen once the conversation actually starts – 'what happens if the patient has a 'bad reaction?' What happens if the patient starts crying – right in the middle of the ward, or in a busy clinic which is already 50 minutes behind time?

Not knowing how to deal with the consequences of what we have begun breaks one of the most fundamental rules of accepted medical behaviour. It makes us inadequate in our own eyes and those of others. There is also the embarrassment of being known as the doctor who goes around making patients cry! It is generally regarded as better for all concerned if dealings with patients go 'smoothly;' and if a patient bursts into tears, many doctors feel that it is because they have failed to do the right things to prevent it. It is not easy to suggest to them that a patient's crying is not in itself a disaster for the doctor or the patient, or that the tears may actually have done the patient some good.

Fear of Expressing Emotion

Doctors are trained to behave calmly in emergencies, suppressing any panic that we may feel; we are also taught to avoid expressing any antagonism that we may feel to an individual patient. These principles are plainly unarguable and central to the accepted idea of proper professional conduct. However, adopting the model of the calm, efficient doctor may lead to the idea that the good doctor does not express *any* emotions. This means that if we wish to express sympathy or other emotion that may be helpful to the patient at the right moment, we have to relearn how to do it.

Doctors are not intrinsically unsympathetic, but having learnt how not to express panic, anger and unhelpful emotions, it becomes a conscious effort to express the sympathy we may naturally feel. I've often heard doctors say how much easier it is to talk to a friend or a neighbour about the way a disease is affecting them, than it is to talk to a patient with the same condition. Perhaps in the clinical setting it's easy to get bogged down by the weight of clinical responsibility and to use authoritative language that disguises both therapeutic failure and underlying sympathy.

There is also an unfortunate semantic quirk that makes this difficulty even worse – and that is the ambiguity of the word 'sorry.' In general use it has two quite distinct meanings. It may be used as in 'I am sorry *that I did this*' which implies responsibility; or it may be used as in 'I am sorry *for you*' to express sympathy. The knack of expressing sympathy and empathy clearly without covertly accepting responsibility, is difficult, and needs to be taught and demonstrated.

Fear of Saying 'I don't Know'

The more junior the doctor the more difficult it is to maintain self confidence while saying 'I don't know.' Perhaps it's the way we are taught to behave in examinations when 'I don't know' is expected to earn failure. In practice, only the most senior and respected doctors are able to earn applause for confessing ignorance. It is almost a universal law that you must be seen to know a very great deal before you are allowed to confess to not knowing it all!

Talking to dying patients may seem at first like taking a examination. It's only after some experience that it becomes apparent that many patients may not want The Answer (and may already know that there isn't one), but may simply want somebody to listen to the problem.

Fear of the Hierarchy

The hierarchical structure of medical and nursing services is essential for the efficient organisation of patient care, but it also means that if a senior doctor (or, less commonly, nurse) decides that patients are not to be told what is wrong with them, it becomes extremely difficult for more junior members to talk freely with the patients. It often happens that juniors are asked by patients whether or not they have cancer, when a senior member has said they are not 'supposed' to know. This is often a very delicate matter and the junior's reluctance to disobey the orders from above makes the patient feel that there is some conspiracy of silence, which is exactly what it is. This will heighten the fears and feelings of isolation in the patient.

Taking Responsibility for the Bad News Itself

If despite all his anxieties and fears, a doctor does begin to talk about the bad news, other factors begin to operate which push him into assuming responsibility for the disease itself. It makes him more and more identifiable as the target for blame, rather than as the ally and supporter of the patient.

Shielding

Some people are more inclined than others to pat a seriously ill patient on the shoulder and reassure him that all will be well. Those who do this most readily are not uncaring, and in fact, the opposite is more likely to be true. They want the news to be good (especially if they have begun to identify with the patient) and they hope that an optimistic picture will hearten the patient. But wishing for a successful outcome doesn't produce it; and by shielding the patient, the doctor removes the opportunity for him to react and behave in his own way to the news, or to take an intelligent part in his own care.

I neither say that shielding should never take place (because roughly half of patients indicate that they would rather not be told the exact diagnosis), nor do I say that every gloomy detail and possible horror must be spelt out. But I believe that shielding should not be a matter of course without even considering the possibility that the patient may want to make up his own mind. If the latter is not accepted, about half of the patients will see the doctor as assuming total command, and some might identify him with the disease instead of with the fight against it.

Taking the Credit for Remission

Talking about the possibility of future relapse is another painful experience, and there is always a great temptation to dismiss it altogether ("we got it in time," "we took it all away"). This is another example of shielding, and patients often overtly encourage us in it, making it difficult not to go along with it. They may be just recovering from primary treatment and be feeling well and optimistic for the first time since diagnosis, and they ask us for encouragement to speed their recovery. It's very easy to agree, even tacitly, that the patient is cured.

The problem is that if a cure is promised in those situations in which relapse is likely, future recurrence will be seen as the personal failure of the doctor. The patient will probably see it that way, and the doctor may also feel, even subconsciously, that the relapse is a failure to fulfil the promise, and he may subsequently avoid contact with the patient for this reason.

Exerting Control over the Information

As mentioned above, our training concentrates on the control of disease processes and it's very frustrating when that can't be achieved. This frustration may lead to a search for some aspect of the situation that can be controlled – and often, this is the information given to the patient and relatives. Exerting control over the information may not alter the clinical prospects but it does offer the chance of behaving in a "doctorly" sort of way. It's very difficult to realise while you are doing it that you may not be helping the patient at all.

What Can Be Done?

I have met many doctors who are good at talking with seriously ill and dying patients, and a few who are absolutely superb at it and from whose example I have learnt a great deal. Only one or two of them, however, have had the time, opportunity and motivation to teach formally or informally on the skills they use, and the principles that guide them. This is sad, because a great amount of accumulated experience goes to waste and it seems almost as if every trainee must learn all the lessons afresh for himself.

I would advocate that medical students receive more detailed instruction and demonstrations in the subject than they do at present. Only by introducing the subject at an early stage will it be seen as part of the orthodox medical curriculum rather than as an esoteric obsession of medical philosophers. In those centres where a course has been set up, it has been shown feasible to integrate it into undergraduate teaching and also to assess the students in the subject.

The most important practical point is that there are many well-known interview techniques which can be of great help. For instance, it is possible to demonstrate the use of open questions to establish how the patient is feeling at the time, and what they know of their disease. Students can be taught how to find out whether or not the patient wants to know more and how to introduce the information. There are well-established facilitation techniques which help patients express their most important worries and anxieties, and students can also be shown how not to react adversely to a patient's anger or need to blame someone. All of these skills have been in use by therapists and counsellors for decades, but medical students are not usually made aware of their value or existence. As regards the methods of teaching, many different media are available. The subjects can be dealt with in lectures, by video programmes, in discussion groups, by role-play under supervision and by interviews with patients.

Conclusion

This chapter has tried to identify the main reasons for our failure to communicate helpfully with patients and relatives about serious illness and dying. In suggesting that this subject be introduced formally into the undergraduate curriculum, I am not proposing major changes in medical teaching or the abandonment of previously held beliefs or standards. I am proposing a change in emphasis which I believe will produce a rapid and noticeable improvement in patient care. Communicating with seriously ill people is a skill, not a gift and it can be taught like any other aspect of medical care. It can be done well by all of us and can give satisfaction when done well. Above all, it should be seen by everyone as a vital part of the job of looking after sick people.

Further Reading

Ahmedzai, S. (1982). Dying in hospital; the resident's viewpoint. British Medical Journal, 285, 712–4.
Bendix, T. (1982). The Anxious Patient. E. & S. Livingstone, London.
Brewin, T.B. (1977). The cancer patient; communication and morale. British Medical Journal, ii, 1623–7.

Buckman, R. (1984). Breaking bad news: why is it still so difficult? British Medical Journal, i, 1597–9.

Goldie, L. (1982). The ethics of telling the patient. Journal of Medical Ethics, 8, 128–33.

Hinton, J. (1972). Dying, Pelican Books, London.

Irwin, W.G. (1984). Teaching terminal care at Queen's University of Belfast. British Medical Journal, ii, 1509–11 & 1604–5.

Jones, S. (1981). Telling the right patient. British Medical Journal, 283, 291–2.

Konior, G.S., Levine, A.S. (1975). Fear of dying: how patients and their doctors behave. Seminars in Oncology, 2, 311–6.

Moreland, C. (1982). Disabilities and how to live with them: testicular teratoma. Lancet, ii, 203–5.

Novack, D.H., Clumer, R., Smith, R.L. et al. (1979). Changes in physicians' attitudes towards telling the patient. American Medical Journal Association, 241, 897–900.

Parkes, C.M. (1978). Psychological aspects. In The Management of Terminal Diseases. (Ed. C.M. Saunders). Arnold, London, p. 44–64.

Sanson-Fisher, R., Maguire, P. (1980). Should skills in communicating with patients be taught in medical schools? Lancet, ii, 523–6

Souhami, R.L. (1978). Teaching what to say about cancer. Lancet, ii, 935–6.

Video Material

Buckman, R., Maguire, P. Why won't they talk to me? An introductory course in communication (5 tapes). Linkward Productions, Shepperton, Herts, England.

Chapter 19

One Patient Looks at Cancer

BRYAN A. SKINNER

This chapter is concerned with one man's perception of his own particular situation. As such, it is a reflection of my own personality, background and experience of cancer, and to a limited extent, what I have learnt directly from friends with cancer.

Details of my background may help in making meaningful comparisons with the situation of others. Some two and a half years ago, at the age of 52, I was diagnosed as having lymphoma – a variant of chronic lymphatic leukaemia. Although this is a disease for which a "cure" is not at present possible, my doctors were hopeful of long periods of remission. Unfortunately, the disease has proved to be rather more aggressive and the remission periods have been limited. Basically, the symptoms are being treated in order to make me as comfortable as possible, and during this two and a half year period I have had three courses of chemotherapy, two of radiotherapy and I am about to commence a further course of treatment.

On the personal front, I am happily married with four grown-up children. In business life, I am a successful entrepreneur and not surprisingly, I am full of stress and anxieties and intolerant of opposition. In the past I have always had abundant drive and energy, but worried about potential problems and made numerous contingency plans for events which, in the main, never occurred. I am a compulsive worker and compulsive about time and achieving objectives, whether they are important or not.

Being told that I had a malignant disease which would shorten my life expectancy was an enormous shock and I felt panic and depression. I had four underlying emotional reactions. The first was a feeling of enormous sadness that I would be leaving my family prematurely, and this applied particularly to my wife. Second, there was a fear of continuously degenerating health with discomfort and possibly pain – I come from a long line of cowards! Third, I had some fear of the unknown – what really does come after death? Fourth, I had a mild feeling of regret that I would not be able to enjoy the fruits of many years of labour.

Before being involved myself, I used to think that friends with cancer were terribly brave. When you suffer the experience, you realise that bravery has nothing to do with the situation. You did not volunteer for the condition; what you need to be is resilient.

Taking a Hand in Your Own Health

I was given the original prognosis as being relatively optimistic, but fifteen months later, the disease was declared to be more aggressive than orginally hoped. At this stage, it became clear that with the best will in the world, the doctors could offer only limited remissions. Given this situation, it was very important for me to make a plan and to feel that I was taking charge of the situation. People like myself who take initiative and responsibility in life, are commonly in fear of flying on aeroplanes, because they have no control over the actual flying of the aeroplane. For such people, taking control of and participating in one's health is important, and the alternative would be fear and despondency, which in itself would be damaging and harmful.

The starting point was to reconsider and assess the quality of medical advice I was receiving. I had been attending a leading oncologist and I had taken advantage of his suggestion to obtain a second opinion from another leading oncologist who confirmed the diagnosis, prognosis and treatment already in hand. So that happily, I had every confidence in the advice and treatment being received. I wondered whether to make a tour of the leading cancer clinics in the USA, but a few written and telephone enquiries revealed that I would simply receive the same treatment. What I did do was to produce a file of my medical records, and if I hear of any clinic or hospital anywhere in the world, which may hold out some hope of a breakthrough, I send them my records and ask if they think they can help. So far I have not received any positive answers but, at least, I feel that I am not leaving these particular stones unturned, while at the same time, I am not wasting my strength struggling around the world.

The second thing I had to do was to reorganise my way of life so that I could be as well, happy and content as possible. I have reached the point where I do those things which I enjoy, and I avoid those which cause me physical discomfort or make me overtired. It is quite fun becoming a caricature of oneself! My family are at pains to make my life as serene as possible and I receive total support from my medical advisers, colleagues and friends. In addition, I make an effort to enjoy every minute of every day. These are the circumstances in which both medical treatment and complementary healing are more likely to succeed. If you organise yourself physically and mentally in this way, it has the clear advantage of improving your quality of life and, hopefully, also the quantity.

In this connection, two points which I have discovered may be helpful to others. First, it is easy to say "enjoy every minute of every day" but when you are suffering from a major disease you often have minor associated ailments which go either with the disease or the treatment. When you add chemotherapy or radiotherapy, there are times when enjoyment and positive thinking are not possible. At those times, I believe it is sufficient not to give in to despair, but to try to build up strength and energy to be able to return to the healing phase. This is where resilience comes in.

These are the times when you need the maximum sympathy, support and tolerance from your close family.

The second point is that the ability to enjoy each day is, in part, a function of how you organise your life. If you are in some physical discomfort or drained of energy, then a day spent chasing around can be agony and probably harmful to your underlying condition. On the other hand, if you spend that day at home in comfort and are able to make running repairs you can probably turn that day into a plus day, i.e. one that is worth living. I score each day a plus or a minus, and with the adjustment of my pattern and attitude of life, minus days are few and far between.

As happens with every cancer patient, various adaptive psychological changes were inevitable. Fundamentally, they all had to do with acceptance and denial – one being the mirror image of the other. Oddly enough, there is evidence that the closer the patient can achieve total or hard core denial, the greater the chances of remission and survival. However, only about one percent of patients are able to maintain denial of this degree to the very end. The weakness of total denial is that if eventually the patient has to face reality he has nothing to fall back on and goes into total despair.

A level of acceptance enables a patient to face up to the disease, the treatments and the prognosis, and still take an active part in his treatment. Acceptance is a mood in which patients may or may not be happy but they are not likely to be terribly sad. Taken to the ultimate stage, acceptance can become resignation, a stage at which most patients require support from only one person and that support is required in the form of help and comfort.

Every cancer patient has to find their own level between denial and resignation. In my case, I could not intellectually refute the diagnosis. This meant that I could not deny that I had the disease, nor, in view of the medical prognosis, could I convince myself that I would definitely recover by medical means. This led me to recognise that I was looking for a miracle – to seek it in a determined manner but to accept that it might not be possible. I therefore decided that I would continue orthodox medical treatment but with the addition of complementary medical therapies in my search for a miracle.

In order to combat the initial panic and depression, the first thing I had to do was to learn to face death as a possibility with a good level of acceptance. Unless I could overcome my fears and emotions it would be difficult for me to address myself to the quality of life and to the prospects of healing. In truth, my anxieties were about death as separation from wife and family, and I needed a defence to take the form of belief or hope of union in death. In the world apporoximately 200,000 people die every day, but most of us shut out death by ignoring it.

There were various things that helped me to adjust. First, I found that reading the books of Elizabeth Kübler-Ross was extremely helpful in the simple acceptance that death is inevitable. That I should not waste my days on earth worrying over this event, but rather that I should concentrate on enjoying each day and thus improve the quality of life – or when it comes, the quality of death. I also know that for me the manner of dying is more important than the timing. I do not wish to die alone in hospital, but at home in the company of my family.

In addition, I received help from the Church. I also visited a leading medium and from the conversations, I can only believe that I was speaking with my father and grandparents who died some time ago. I am convinced that I have a soul which will survive after life on earth, that I am on this world for a purpose, that I will meet my family and friends in the next world and that after death, all will be revealed.

Once I had arrived at this point in acceptance of death I was in a position to look for my "miracle." Unfortunately, there are no classes on this subject and I had to evolve my own plan. Even a little research will reveal that miracles or spontaneous remissions can and do occur at any stage in the progress of a cancer, even after last rites have been administered. Therefore, there is always hope and the search is worthwhile.

A Search for Self-Help

When I decided to try self-help I found that there was a considerable volume of literature, tapes and lectures available. Unfortunately, much of this is contradictory and confusing. The confusion arises for two main reasons. First, many approaches to self healing are an 'act of faith' – and that is meant both with and without religious connotations. We are considering techniques which work for some people without a scientific explanation being available. Second, many of the books are written from an over-committed and blinkered viewpoint. In terms of logic, they attempt the impossible by formulating categorical propositions from situations which cannot be accurately described in a perfectly unambiguous manner.

In order to arrive at a reasoned approach to self-healing, it helps to view it as being more related to philosophy than to science. Philosophical hypotheses are based on experience, and are intended to explain experience; that is different from being capable of confirmation or confutation by observation or experiment under specified conditions. The scientific hypotheses (orthodox medicine) must not only account for all the observations already made of the phenomenon concerned, but must be capable of being definitely confirmed or confuted by further observations or experiments under specified conditions.

The medical approach to getting well is the scientific approach, whereas self-help or "healing" is the philosophical approach or the act of faith. It is my belief that the two are complementary and I would not wish to ignore either approach by pursuing one to the exclusion of the other. Many of the books on alternative medicine loose credibility, because they deprecate orthodox medicine and because they try to provide a scientific or logical explanation where none exists.

Given this background and the fact that I was in unchartered waters, I felt it was important to obtain a medical view of any complementary medical approach I was considering. I examine medical advice similarly. I regard advice which I receive from the doctor (or elsewhere) not as instruction but advice, and *advice* is something to be considered while decisions are to be taken by the person concerned. This is particularly true in the case of cancer where treatment may be controversial. It was essential for me to participate in the decisions because the act of participation (my agreement) could well affect the outcome of the particular treatment.

It has not been scientifically proven how far the mind can influence the immune system or other body processes in order to cure or gain remission from cancer. Since there was no scientific proof, I had to develop my own philosophical approach based on the evidence available, and decide whether a particular technique appealed to me. One of the great things about complementary medicine is that you can select those techniques with no harmful potential.

The techniques of self-help which I have found useful are first, to improve my attitude of mind and to try to eliminate harmful negative emotions. The second is relaxation and the third visualisation. There are various approaches to each of these and they are well covered in various books (see List of Reading).

Apart from self-help I also decided to visit healers. Before becoming involved, my basic attitude was that I accepted that healing took place but on a very, very infrequent basis. I was extremely fortunate that on my first visit to the Harry Edwards Healing Sanctuary, I witnessed a remarkable cure (not of cancer, unfortunately). Subsequent reading of books by Harry Edwards and Tom Pilgrim convinced me that although it was only in a minority of cases, nevertheless a significant number of cures were effected by healers. My own conclusions about healing are as follows:

1. Accept that healing may occur but is not certain. It would be unreasonable to expect more than this, if only because most people go to healers when the medical profession cannot provide a cure. Further if all healing was successful we would have no need of doctors.

2. Be relaxed during the healing sessions so that you do not resist healing, and be positive in your approach to healing and the prospects. The effectiveness of healing can be affected by the subconscious mind which can reject the suggestion by the conscious mind. This is why the physical stimulus which is part of regular contact healing, can be important. In the laying-on of hands, the physical reality can be sensed by the subconscious of the subject and helps it to accept the suggestion.

3. When you pray for healing you should ask for healing "if it is God's will."

4. For most serious diseases, healing is more likely to occur gradually rather than immediately, and instant cures are few and far between. In the case of arthritis and similar complaints, dramatic results appear more common.

5. Obtain healing on a regular and frequent basis so that if you have to travel,

visit leading healers wherever you go. I feel that all the sources of healing work together and I do not make comparisons, although some healers are better at dealing with certain complaints than others.

Some people may have to open their minds and re-examine certain orthodox teachings and established attitudes. They may have been taught that such matters are to be regarded as some sort of mental aberration. Some religions are against healing and others only accept those within the Church – and by that they mean *their* Church. I can only suggest that the bigotry, prejudices, creeds, dogmas and trivialities which constitute orthodoxy, are manmade, whereas the universe is God-given.

I felt that I also had to give consideration to the subject of diet, I must admit that the idea of taking masses of carrot juice and the like did not appeal, and I would therefore have required very strong evidence before altering my eating habits in any material way. I asked, separately, two leading cancer consultants for their advice. In their view, there is no evidence to suggest that these diets have any beneficial effects, whilst at the same time they could reduce the quality of life. I found this also to be the view of a number of doctors who are involved in complementary medicine. There is positive opposition to the extreme diets and enema treatments, such as those recommended by Gerson.

In addition, the cost is significant and the time to purchase and prepare the food, etc. can be a full-time job for one person. It struck me that this was a subject capable of scientific appraisal in the same way as treatment by drugs, and therefore I was prepared to follow the view of the vast majority of medical practitioners spoken to, and simply pursue a balanced diet.

One of the problems in such an enquiry is to decide where complementary medicine ends and quackery begins. There are dozens of so called "cures" from laetrile to mistletoe, and some persist throughout the World, but I could find no agency in the UK from which to obtain a balanced view of their trials and research. In the United States the Cancer Information Service examines and reports on some 2,500 "cures" a year for cancer! No wonder the UK patient is confused and is often ready to try almost any remedy as a last resort.

I thought of attending one of the alternative medicine cancer clinics in Mexico, located there because they are prohibited by law in the United States. On checking with several sources, including medical practitioners in the USA who believe in complementary medicine, I decided against this course. The reports were generally unfavourable, including reports of people who had been told they were cured and then found by their physician to have active cancer on returning home.

There is a dilemma in how much time and attention one should give to getting well. You wish to get well and put the disease behind you, but can you do that when you are spending most of your time and attention thinking about and treating you condition? Are you in fact creating tensions and feeding your disease? Is this one reason why the hard core denial people do well compared with others? It all depends on the basic personality of the individual. In every day life I cannot put a praoblem behind me if it exists, and I worry most about problems I cannot get round to dealng with. Therefore, since leukaemia is my biggest problem in life, I am most comfortable about it when I am actively doing something about the problem. For me, the best situation is to feel that I am leaving no stone unturned, but this approach may be inappropriate for others.

I have one friend who finds difficulty in the apparent contradiction of accepting that the statistical odds are that you will die of you disease, and yet you are fighting to recover. I have no problems with this on the basis that when you know and accept the worse, you can then put it behind you and proceed with trying to get well.

My Conclusions on Support Therapies Are as Follows:
1. They can improve the quality of life, and I feel that this is beyond doubt. This in itself makes them worthwhile.
2. They achieve this by encouraging a positive approach.
3. The positive approach arises from: (a) acceptance of death (b) providing a ray of hope – in the last resort, inexplicable remissions, however infrequent or unlikely, do occur. In general I would accept a therapy if it might work and does no harm. This is sufficient to give hope (c) counterbalancing the wilder form of alternative medicine propaganda, depressing or worrying advice and situations (d) learning how to deal with low periods (e) enabling patients to participate in their own health.
4. I believe that it is possible in certain cases to extend the period of valuable life or to influence the course of the disease. There is no unequivocal evidence of this and the proposition is hypothetical.
5. It is conceivable that remission and cures can be brought about by a positive approach combined with healing. Again a hypothetical proposition.

Personal Relationships

Few problems arise with friends and business acquaintances. Once people understood the importance of helping me to avoid infections and not overtire myself, they have been kindness itself. One of the strange things with leukaemia, particularly if you are taking steroids, is that you tend to look very well and a few people have difficulty in understanding the nature and seriousness of your disease. The result is that these people continue to impose pressures and strains which can drain your much needed energy. You must be quick to recognise these people and act accordingly.

One of the nicest aspects is the interest and kindness of people I hardly know. Two of the most frequently used phrases by such people are "my wife and I are not very religious but we will pray for you,'' and ''I pray for you every day.'' People also go out of their way to contact me to let me know that if I have to conduct some business anywhere in the world, they will do it for me. Such things give me a very warm glow inside.

Particularly in the period following diagnosis, I would receive information every day from some friend about a new cure, treatment or clinic. None of these proved positive but they were useful background information helping me to complete an overall picture. However, one thing I find rather irritating is when people with no knowledge say ''they can cure your disease these days'' or otherwise claim to know someone with your condition who was cured some years ago. Whenever I have followed up any of these, I have found either that they had something different or that they were not cured. I know that I should not be irritated bacause people are only trying to provide hope – but this is counter-productive unless it has some worthwhile basis.

One factor which has been beneficial in my case is that I have a good friend who has cancer. We share our knowledge, experience and experiments and this is mutually beneficial. We also laugh a lot when we are together and this is beneficial.

Some families and individuals feel they do not want other people to know they have cancer. This attitude is totally wrong because you need all the understanding and help you can get. Most of the help you are going to need has to come from your family, your doctors and the healers. However, from your colleagues, friends and acquaintances you need understanding. If they know of your conditon you will be amazed at the genuine level of concern.

In this connection I well remember that some years ago I was at odds with a business colleague because I did not think his mind was on the business. Unfortunately, his wife was terminally ill with cancer and he had chosen not to tell anyone. I have always regretted adding to the man's burden, particularly as he had his priorities right. Had he informed me of the circumstances, I could have been helpful and understanding instead of an additional burden.

Equally, it is important to be careful how you use sympathy. Cancer is a powerful solver. You get your emotional needs met, you gain sympathy, love and attention. It allows people to give up on various things, or choose what they want to do. This can be an advantage or a disadvantage. You should use this experience to improve the quality and enjoyment of life and this then becomes a positive factor. What you should not do is to use the attention in a negative way so that subconsciously you wish to remain ill and retain the attention.

You have to be wary of the psychological approach to the cause of cancer. We can all accept that there are certain personality types likely to be more prone to cancer or any other illness (e.g. Type 'A' Heart personalities). Qualities that are likely to cause people to be successes in life could possibly contribute to suppressing the immune system and allow disease to progress. However, the suggestion that psychosocial factors may predispose to cancer may make you feel that you have caused your own disease and this would work against your self healing. Again, you do need a psychiatrist to deal with your normal moods because they are the characteristic patterns of response to be expected of a cancer patient. Your close family has to understand your attitudes and it should not take too much effort.

One thing I came to realise early on was that there were two people deeply affected by my disease – my wife and myself. This situation calls for mutual support. As a patient you have to realise that anger, irritability and grief must be hard to bear by the spouse looking after the patient, although there is a case to be made out for the patient to sometimes let go of his emotions. The really important factor is to give something back in the relationship and not develop into a "taker." I try to make it clear by every means possible that the love and care is fully understood and reciprocated, and that it is that very relationship which gives me such pleasure in life despite the underlying circumstances. This way we sustain each other and gain great joy.

With regard to medical advisers, I have been extremely fortunate. In such a situation the family doctor is the lynch pin for the patient. On the whole, I have found my medical advisors receptive to complementary medicine and I think that any concern that they may have is with some of the practitioners of complementary medicine rather than with the concept itself.

While I have received every kindness from specialists treating me, there is no time for effective discussion and counselling. I believe that we require counsellors to work with oncologists and perform this service. In the United States there is an excellent organisation called the Cancer Information Service which produces valuable patient literature on the various forms of cancer and their treatments. They also have a telephone enquiry service. A similar service in Britain has currently become available (BACUP).

A considerable amount of time would be saved by doctors with the use of pre-printed communications. Some of the areas to be covered would be:

- Medication direction form – name of medication, dosage, times of day, before and after meals, compatible with alcohol plus any special instructions.

- Possible side effects, how to cope with them, critical levels and any cut-off points. Possible other associated ailments likely to arise – shingles, thrush etc.

- Pre-printed details of possible emotional complications relating to personality types and particular groups – children, adolescents, over-anxious or depressed patients.

- Advice on diet, exercise, sex, climate, sun, travel, post-remission follow-up etc.

- Advice for parents – what to look for and do, when to run for help.

What Should we Offer the Cancer Patient?

How can we offer cancer patients the opportunity to participate in their own health care? I would like to see cancer clinics which would combine the very best of conventional medical treatment coupled with complementary medicine. They must aim at a high standard of excellence in both fields. In the absence of such clinics at present, many patients feel that they have to choose between conventional and alternative medicine, and this in itself gives rise to many problems. This type of clinic would meet the needs of those who wish to explore the possibilities of both types of healing.

The clinics' activities would be centered on the whole patient and should provide patients with the maximum help and the opportunity to participate in their own health. One of the essential features would be to staff the clinics with people who display the qualities of compassion and selflessness. This should apply as much to the junior domestic staff as to the senior consultants. On the medical side, one would need the involvement of leading oncologists in touch with world advances, and in a position to give the best advice available. The aims of the complementary therapies would be to improve the patient's quality of life and possibly extend the period of useful life. The techniques to be used would include counselling, group therapy, relaxation, healing and spiritual support.

What is needed is to create five situations:

- An atmosphere where patients, family and friends can come and discuss their situation, emotions, attitudes etc. in a totally open manner. The aim should be to build a relationship of mutual respect and open communication.

- To have available a range of proven therapies which patients can feel free to follow or reject.

- To give guidance on "treatments" which are considered to be quackery and which can be harmful to the body and/or the pocket.

- To help patients in the acceptance of death. This would necessitate the availability of support, on an inter faith basis, to help in the spiritual understanding of suffering and death so that the patients need not fear that they are to disappear into a black hole. For most people acceptance of death is a prerequisite for taking a positive approach to living and healing.

- To enable patients to participate in their own health.

In summary, these would be cancer centres offering a range of treatments. In purely scientific terms some of the therapies could be described as being experimental, since although it would be accepted that they can improve the quality of life, there is no scientific way of proving that they affect the cancer growth.

Such cancer centres could provide other services too. Literature would be available to give guidance and help to patients about their disease and its management. Local volunteer support groups would emerge who would provide such services as: (a) work in the clinic, (b) transport of patients, (c) raise money to assist patients in financial need, (d) make visits to patients where family support is not available.

Conclusion

Although every individual is likely to react in an unique way, broad patterns of psychological response can be recognised to the diagnosis and progress of cancer and to its treatment. Every patient should be psychologically assessed at the outset in order to identify when problems are likely to arise and how best to deal with then and head them off. Equally, it is necessary to identify sources of strength and how best to utilise these. Out of this will come therapies which will affect the quality of life and may possibly affect the outcome of the disease in that patient.

Fundamentally, for most patients, we have to encourage a positive attitude. In this connection many patients can accept reality as long as there is a ray of hope and confidence that their advisors will not give them up. Without that ray of hope, despair is likely to set in and this can be destructive. Support therapies need to complement the patient's resources and life situation, but the emphasis on particular therapies will vary from individual to individual.

During the "cancer experience" it is possible for a patient not merely to adjust but also to enhance quality of life, achieve personal growth and development and an improved ability to cope with life. They can learn to live in the present rather than in the future, with the greater daily fulfilment which that brings. They are likely to allow time to seek pleasure and gratification in personal relationships and other fields, and may find that they are meeting their true personal needs for the first time. To achieve this aim, patients need help.

Useful Reading Material

1. Getting well again, by Carl Simonton M.D., ISBN 0.553,231480/Bantam Books
2. All about cancer – A practical guide to cancer care by Chris Williams, ISBN 0.471.90037.0/John Wiley & Sons Limited
3. Healng and mind power by Richard Shames, M.D. and Chuck Sterms M.S. Ph.D., ISBN 9.87857.293.7/Rodale Press
4. The dynamic laws of self healing, by Catherine Ponder, ISBN 87516.156.1/De Vorss
5. A manual of self healing, by E.H. Shattock, ISBN 0.85500.169.0/Turnstone Press Limited
6. The secret science at work, by Max Freedom Long, De Vorss
7. The power of spiritual healing, by Harry Edwards, The Healer Publishing Co., Burrows Lea, Shere, Guildford, Surrey.
8. Tom Pilgrim: Autobiography of a spiritual healer by Tom Pilgrim, ISBN 0.7221.6868.2/Sphere Books Limited
9. On death and dying, by Elizabeth Kübler-Ross, ISBN 0.422.75490.0/Tavistock Publications.
10. Death: The final stage of growth, by Elizabeth Kübler-Ross, ISBN 0.13.196998.6/Prentice-Hall.

Index